T0227166

Education

Guest Editor

JANE C. ROTHROCK, DNSc, RN, CNOR, FAAN

PERIOPERATIVE NURSING CLINICS

www.periopnursing.theclinics.com

Consulting Editor
NANCY GIRARD, PhD, RN, FAAN

June 2009 • Volume 4 • Number 2

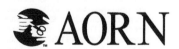

SAUNDERS an imprint of ELSEVIER, Inc.

W.B. SAUNDERS COMPANY

A Division of Elsevier Inc.

1600 John F. Kennedy Boulevard • Suite 1800 • Philadelphia, Pennsylvania 19103-2899

http://www.periopnursing.theclinics.com

PERIOPERATIVE NURSING CLINICS Volume 4, Number 2
June 2009 ISSN 1556-7931, ISBN-13: 978-1-4377-0523-2, ISBN-10: 1-4377-0523-5

Editor: Katie Hartner
Developmental Editor: Donald Mumford

The ideas and opinions expressed in *Perioperative Nursing Clinics* do not necessarily reflect those of the Publisher nor the Association of periOperative Registered Nurses (AORN, Inc). Neither the Publisher nor AORN Inc assume any responsibility for any injury and/or damage to persons or property arising out of or related to any use of the material contained in this periodical. The reader is advised to check the appropriate medical literature and the product information currently provided by the manufacturer of each drug to be administered to verify the dosage, the method and duration of administration, or contraindications. It is the responsibility of the treating physician or other health care professional, relying on independent experience and knowledge of the patient, to determine drug dosages and the best treatment for the patient. Mention of any product in this issue should not be construed as endorsement by the contributors, editors, AORN Inc, or the Publisher of the product or manufacturers' claims. The content of this issue has not been peer reviewed by AORN Inc, and AORN Inc makes no representation as to compliance of the content with the AORN Inc standards, recommended practices or guidelines. AORN's endorsement of the publication does not constitute endorsement of any representations or assertions in the content.

Perioperative Nursing Clinics (ISSN 1556-7931) is published quarterly by Elsevier, 360 Park Avenue South, New York, NY 10010. Months of issue are March, June, September and December. Business and Editorial Offices: 1600 John F. Kennedy Blvd., Suite 1800, Philadelphia, PA 19103-2899. Customer Service Office: 11830 Westline Industrial Drive, St. Louis, MO 63146. Periodicals postage paid at New York, NY and at additional mailing offices. Subscription prices are $116.00 per year (domestic individuals), $209.00 per year (domestic institutions), $58.00 per year (domestic students/residents), $116.00 per year (Canadian individuals), $240.00 per year (Canadian institutions), $150.00 per year (international individuals), $240 per year (international institutions), and $62.00 per year (International and Canadian students/residents). Foreign air speed delivery is included in all *Clinics* subscription prices. All prices are subject to change without notice. **POSTMASTER:** Send change of address to *Perioperative Nursing Clinics*, Customer Service (orders, claims, online, change of address): Elsevier Periodicals Customer Service, 11830 Westline Industrial Drive, St. Louis, MO 63146. Tel: 1-800-654-2452 (U.S. and Canada). Fax: 314-523-5170. E-mail: journalscustomerservice-usa@elsevier.com (for print support); journalsonlinesupport-usa@elsevier.com (for online support).

Reprints. For copies of 100 or more, of articles in this publication, please contact the Commercial Rights Department, Elsevier Inc., 360 Park Avenue South, New York, NY 10010-1710; phone: (+1) 212-633-3813; fax: (+1) 212-462-1935; e-mail: reprints@elsevier.com.

Printed and bound in the United Kingdom
Transferred to Digital Print 2011

Contributors

CONSULTING EDITOR

NANCY GIRARD, PhD, RN, FAAN
Consultant, Boerne; and Clinical Associate Professor, Acute Nursing Care Department, University of Texas Health Science Center, San Antonio, Texas

GUEST EDITOR

JANE C. ROTHROCK, DNSc, RN, CNOR, FAAN
Director of Perioperative Programs, Delaware County Community College, Media, Pennsylvania

AUTHORS

LANA M. DeRUYTER, PhD, RN
Dean, Allied Health and Nursing, Nursing Department, Delaware County Community College, Media, Pennsylvania

DEBRA L. FAWCETT, RN, PhD
Assistant Professor of Nursing, School of Nursing, Indiana University Kokomo, Kokomo, Indiana

BETH FITZGERALD, RN, MSN, CNOR
Perioperative Nurse Internship Manger, Christiana Care Health System, Wilmington, Delaware; Perioperative Instructor, Delaware County Community College, Media, Pennsylvania; and Perioperative Instructor, University of Delaware, Newark, Delaware

NANCY GIRARD, PhD, RN, FAAN
Clinical Associate Professor, Department of Acute Nursing Care, University of Texas Health Science Center at San Antonio, San Antonio, Texas; and Consulting Editor, Perioperative Nursing Clinics, Philadelphia, Pennsylvania

MELANIE O. LEROY, PhD, RN, CRNP
Assistant Professor of Nursing, Nursing Department, Delaware County Community College, Media, Pennsylvania

PATRICIA LOSITO, RN, MSN, ANP
Coordinator, Nursing Department, Erie Community College, State University of New York, Williamsville, New York

JANICE A. NEIL, RN, PhD
Associate Professor, East Carolina University, Greenville, North Carolina

CAROL R. RITCHIE, MSN, RN, CNOR
Clinical Educator, Perioperative Services Scottsdale Healthcare, Scottsdale, Arizona

JANE C. ROTHROCK, DNSc, RN, CNOR, FAAN
Director of Perioperative Programs, Delaware County Community College, Media,
Pennsylvania

ROSE SEAVEY, RN, BS, MBA, CNOR, CRCST
President and CEO, Seavey Healthcare Consulting, Inc., Arvada, Colorado

CHRISTINE E. SMITH, RN, MSN, CNOR
Perioperative Clinical Nurse Specialist, Lucile Packard Children's Hospital at Stanford,
Palo Alto, California

KATHERINE M. ZULICK, BA
Mount Holyoke College, South Hadley, Massachusetts

P. ALAN ZULICK, ESQUIRE, BA, JD
Member, Pennsylvania and Montgomery Bar Associations; Former Chief Counsel,
Pennsylvania Department of General Services; and Trial and Administrative Disciplinary
Law, Media, Pennsylvania

Contents

Clinical placement in nursing education is an emerging and pressing challenge, with the need to expose students to a wide range of positive and
fundamental learning experiences. Employers expect new graduates to
have higher levels of competence, with varied skills and a sharpened ability to think critically. Using perioperative practice settings as clinical sites
can provide an extensive array of learning experiences for nursing students that enhance the knowledge, skills, and values needed to practice
premier nursing at that expected and higher level. This article demonstrates the transferability of skills, knowledge, and values that new graduates can learn in the operating room and provides an overview of how
a clinical operating room experience can help nurse educators achieve
end-of-program outcomes.

In order for perioperative nurses to form educational partnerships with
colleges of nursing, it is helpful for them to understand the culture of the
academic setting. Each academic setting is unique in its curricular design.
In order for perioperative nurses to collaborate effectively with the
academic institution in fostering its curricular outcomes, it is necessary
to understand the beliefs of the faculty regarding nursing and nursing practice. This article focuses on the nursing curriculum at a community college
and the objectives and integration of an observational experience in perioperative patient care.

Clinical simulation is rapidly becoming important in nursing education.
Nursing faculty members are challenged to prepare nurses for complex
environments and work with interdisciplinary teams. In addition, health
care administrators expect basic competence from new nursing graduates. The new generation of nursing students is often video and computer
savvy, and case studies and computer interactive CDs may not be as
effective with this generation. Although more research is needed on
high-fidelity simulation, it can be an exciting application of advanced technology in nursing education. It is rapidly becoming state-of-the-art in

nursing education because it can bridge the gap between classroom instruction and the unpredictable clinical area.

Creating a place for perioperative nursing in graduate programs can be challenging but rewarding for the hospital, student, and instructor. Adding perioperative content into an existing academic program is possible, and doing so allows students to focus on their chosen specialty. A higher education degree, such as a master's degree in nursing or a doctorate, benefits the nurse. Ultimately, nurses who attain higher education degrees benefit every health care institution in which they serve.

This article discusses the results of two studies, with the first focused on baccalaureate students and registered nurses and the second focused on associate degree nursing students, identifying their culture, care, education, and experiences. Improving the number of graduating African-American nursing students has the potential to advance workforce diversity. Minority students who graduate from nursing programs and who then seek advanced degrees to educate future nurses contribute two-fold: improving diversity among nurse educators and providing minority students with more and important ethnic role models within the nursing profession.

To provide the highest-quality health care to its people, the United States must overcome the communication gap between those who have low health literacy levels or low English proficiency levels and the level of health literacy required to navigate the health care system. Effective communication with patients and the delivery of safe, equitable, and quality care are underpinned by issues of responding to diversity, culture, language, and health literacy. The changes suggested in this article are not only practical ways to improve the quality of health care for all Americans but are also sound economic proposals that in the end will promote the well-being of patients, providers, and even insurers if these initiatives are actively and fully pursued.

At the Christiana Care Health System (CCHS), novice perioperative nurses have the opportunity to make the transition from novice to advanced beginner in a supportive environment where they can build their skills under the supervision and guidance of a qualified educator and dedicated preceptors. A perioperative internship program has been tailored to meet the needs of the facility and ensures novice nurses acquire a strong didactic and clinical foundation using evidence-based practices. CCHS perioperative services have developed their own successful perioperative internship program to address the nursing shortage in its perioperative settings.

Developing Simulation Scenarios for Perioperative Nursing Core Competencies and Patient Safety

Christine E. Smith

The perioperative environment is highly complex and technologically dense, makes use of interdisciplinary teams, and relies on human factors. These characteristics make the perioperative environment rich in opportunities to practice, test, investigate, and validate patient-care processes. Every process and procedure of this environment pose risks for patients and present chances of errors. For perioperative nurses preparing for this workplace, active learning exercises in a clinically realistic setting can improve psychomotor performance, critical-thinking decision making, clinician confidence, professional satisfaction, and interpersonal team skills. Simulation scenario training for the perioperative setting is a valuable educational tool for educating clinicians, for meeting regulatory expectations, and for promoting patient and staff safety.

Fundamental Perioperative Nursing: Decompartmentalizing the Scrub and Circulator Roles

Carol R. Ritchie

Historically, operating room nurses served in the scrub and circulator roles. Today registered nurses predominantly circulate and the scrub role has been delegated to surgical technologists. While the registered nurse may no longer routinely take on the scrub role, he or she needs to be comfortable and confident delegating and supervising the scrub person. In our setting, many registered nurses in perioperative were not comfortable in the role of scrub person. A scrub fellowship for registered Nurses was developed by Scottsdale Healthcare and collaborators to encourage the RN to have more involvement in the scrub role. The scrub fellowship program teaches experienced perioperative nurses how to scrub on the majority of high-volume procedures in their specialty unit. Scrubbing increases the perioperative nurse's knowledge about procedures and provides direct experience and appreciation of activities at the sterile field. This gives the nurse greater competence at delegating the role, a learned skill that requires experience as well as effective communication. Furthermore, the experience in the scrub role improves the nurse's ability to identify and speak up about potential patient safety concerns at the sterile field, and gives the perioperative nurse confidence and competence to supervise the person assigned to the scrub role.

Sterile processing (SP) plays a vital role in patient safety. With ever-changing technology in surgical instrumentation, sterilization/disinfection methods, and monitoring, there is an increasing need for staff well educated in SP. Health care facilities need a standardized orientation program and consistent, on-going educational programs designed specifically for SP. Mandatory certification for SP professionals is a highly recommended, laudatory goal.

THE CLINICS ARE NOW AVAILABLE ONLINE!

Access your subscription at:
www.theclinics.com

Preface

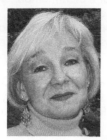

Jane C. Rothrock, DNSc, RN, CNOR, FAAN
Guest Editor

Education—President Obama is increasing the budget for it, college administrators are trying to measure its outcomes, surgical services directors are seeking creative ways to deliver it, undergraduate nursing students are fretting over whether it will help them pass the National Council Licensure Examination, and perioperative nurses are looking for educational options that meet their own clinical interests. It has been my unique privilege to collaborate with a number of experts in bringing you this issue with its multi-faceted focus on education. Educating perioperative nurses for entry-level practice and for expanded roles as first assistants has been my life's work. Even so, I found each of the perspectives in the articles in this issue of the *Perioperative Nursing Clinics* refreshing, unique, helpful, and current. I am confident that you will too.

The publication of the Association of periOperative Registered Nurses'[1] guidance statement on the "Value of clinical learning activities in undergraduate nursing curricula" revitalized discussions of how to incorporate perioperative clinical assignments and rotations in nursing programs. We know that lack of nursing faculty in general is a primary reason for the inability of nursing programs to increase enrollments (American Association of Colleges of Nursing).[2] A review of strategies to address the nursing faculty shortage suggests that educational partnerships can be collaborative efforts that add clinical sites.[3] This issue includes articles that look at perioperative experiences in undergraduate and graduate nursing education and reviews the use of simulation in that education.

The complex issues of diversity and health literacy are fundamental in educating nurses and patients. The authors of the article on diversity in nursing education undertook their studies for their doctoral dissertations. I hope more doctoral students undertake similar studies, helping us all generalize findings to any of our educational endeavors. Health literacy, an essential concept for patient education, is presented with an informative legal analysis of the relationship between the process of informed consent and health literacy. This should help the reader understand both of these critical processes.

Clinical educators will find four intriguing and interesting articles. They address: (1) the preparation of novice perioperative nurses, (2) a scrub fellowship for experienced perioperative nurses, (3) the development and use of simulation scenarios in clinical

Perioperative Nursing Clinics 4 (2009) xi–xii
doi:10.1016/j.cpen.2009.03.001
1556-7931/09/$ – see front matter © 2009 Published by Elsevier Inc.

education, and (4) the education of staff in central processing. Each of these articles offers practical applications and useful information.

Every time you educate a patient, a nursing student, or a staff member, you allow another "flower" to bloom. I fully hope that we will be able to harvest those "flowers" you nurtured and encourage them to write about their experiences in the *Perioperative Nursing Clinics*, increasing the harvest of good ideas, lessons learned, and emerging best practices.

Jane C. Rothrock, DNSc, RN, CNOR, FAAN
Delaware County Community College
901 South Media Line Road
Media, PA 19063, USA

E-mail address:
jrothrock@dccc.edu (J.C. Rothrock)

REFERENCES

1. Value of perioperative clinical learning activities in undergraduate nursing curricula. In: Perioperative standards and recommended practices. Denver: The Association; 2009. p. 289–92.
2. 2007–2008 Enrollment and graduations in baccalaureate and graduate programs in nursing. www.aacn.nche.edu/IDS/datarep.htm. Accessed February 1, 2009.
3. Allan JD, Aldebron J. A systematic assessment of strategies to address the nursing faculty shortage. US Nursing Outlook 2008;56:286–97.

Using the Operating Room to Meet End-of-Program Outcomes

Debra L. Fawcett, RN, PhD

KEYWORDS

- Education • Perioperative • End-of-program outcomes
- Clinical

One of the most challenging issues for nursing today is the recruitment and education of sufficient numbers of nursing professionals to meet health care needs. The good news is that continuing efforts to boost enrollment in schools of nursing have increased the numbers of students. The bad news is that currently there is not enough nursing faculty to educate those numbers. The National League of Nursing reported that 18% of qualified candidates applying for nursing school had to be turned away for lack of qualified faculty.[1]

Not only are inadequate faculty numbers a problem, but quality clinical sites for the nursing student's education remain in short supply in the face of increasing enrollments. Competition for clinical sites is a growing concern. Schools and faculty seek clinical sites that offer diverse opportunities for skill development, decision making, and critical thinking. Long standing partnerships offer some schools units with a wide range of opportunities but cannot accommodate an increase in numbers of students or in other schools. Add to that the pressure on hospitals to provide clinical sites for students in respiratory therapy, x-ray, licensed practical nursing students, and surgical technology and what emerges is acute stress for already overburdened staff nurses and potential stiff competition for the clinical sites available to the nursing education program.

Since the 1950s, there has been a net decline in the number of nursing programs that offer perioperative nursing as part of their curricula.[2,3] The subsequent decrease has led to a severe shortage of available new graduates with perioperative nursing experience across America. Most nursing programs only offer a one day observational experience in the OR. In select nursing education programs where there is qualified faculty, an elective experience in perioperative patient care may be offered. The rich

School of Nursing, Indiana University Kokomo, 2300 South Washington Street, P.O. Box 9003, Kokomo, IN 46902, USA

E-mail address: debra.fawcett@wishard.edu

Perioperative Nursing Clinics 4 (2009) 79–85
doi:10.1016/j.cpen.2009.01.007
1556-7931/09/$ – see front matter © 2009 Elsevier Inc. All rights reserved.

opportunities offered in a perioperative clinical rotation are rarely fully recognized, however, in nursing education programs.

In 2008, more nursing education programs have begun to view perioperative clinical sites, such as an acute care operating room (OR) setting or the ambulatory surgery setting, and the opportunities they offer for clinical experience in a new light. To maintain this positive momentum, both perioperative nurse clinicians and nurse educators need to understand the opportunities offered by a clinical experience in the operating room. The knowledge, skills, and values available for learning in the OR are exceptional. Indeed, many of the opportunities can be transferred to the very foundation of nursing and used in any setting whether it is a clinic, office, outpatient surgical center, or ICU.

TRANSFERABILITY OF KNOWLEDGE

Perioperative practice takes place in many arenas and not just in the acute care OR. Principles learned and practiced in the OR and its associated areas can be applied in any practice sphere. Some skills and values learned while working with the perioperative patient include verification of procedures, informed consent, communication, and assessment. Each of these skills is used daily in the OR and most are used multiple times. Patient safety has taken center stage as a key issue over the past years and must be observed in every health care setting. Verification of surgical procedures and identification of the patient is a primary step toward a safe patient environment. Where else is informed consent used for every procedure and checked by multiple levels of caregivers before the surgical procedure can go forward? Students are sometimes afraid to communicate with physicians, but an experience in the OR often requires the student to work one-on-one with anesthesiologists and surgeons and with the rest of the surgical team, diminishing the fear to communicate with physicians and enabling students to work efficiently and effectively. Students are also allowed the opportunity to report laboratory values and patient conditions directly to the team, thereby teaching the value of clear, concise communication. All areas of nursing practice ultimately require these communication skills.

The principle of asepsis is a fundamental cornerstone of all nursing practice; it is practiced, taught, learned, and integrated within all perioperative practice settings. The critical principles of asepsis can be applied to most areas of nursing practice to prevent infection (**Figs. 1** and **2**). Principles of asepsis are used when putting in a Foley

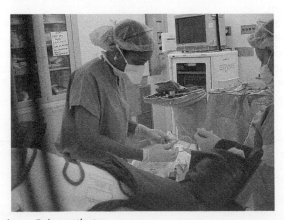

Fig. 1. Nurse inserting a Foley catheter.

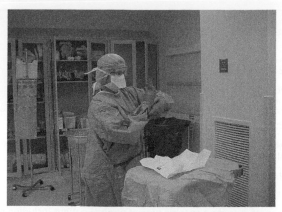

Fig. 2. Nurse putting on sterile gloves.

catheter, changing a dressing, assisting with a Pik line, and in the significantly important practice of hand washing.

Teamwork is a hallmark of perioperative nursing practice and an essential element of collaboration and patient safety. Each member of the surgical team has a responsibility to work with other members to provide a safe and positive outcome for the patient. In the OR, each team member must participate in procedures to verify correct procedures, correct site surgery, patient identification procedures, and patient safety issues. Teamwork, both in the OR and other areas of patient care, is an overarching factor in patient safety.

Important values are also inherent in the practice of perioperative patient care. Each patient deserves the right to privacy. It is the responsibility of the surgical team to provide privacy for the surgical patient and to demonstrate respect for that privacy by keeping the patient covered as much as possible and by making sure unnecessary people are not going in and out of the OR room. The name of the patient, the procedure performed, and other patient information are kept confidential; what an excellent place to understand the rationale behind HIPPA guidelines and to practice them.

Nurses must become patient advocates during surgical procedures because the patient is often unconscious or under the effects of sedative medications and unable to speak for themselves. The surgical team also recognizes the patient as a person and not just a procedure. Students learn invaluable sensitivity and observe first

---

Box 1
Sophomore level outcomes communication

Outcome

Identify therapeutic communication techniques

Learning experiences

Follow perioperative nurse while doing preoperative assessment, team communication

Assignments

Report on communication techniques during postconference

Write a paper explaining how the nurse used therapeutic communication

> **Box 2**
> **Junior level outcomes communication**
>
> *Outcome*
> Use of therapeutic communication in specific client situations
>
> *Learning experiences*
> Review of policies related to discharge teaching
> Do discharge teaching to a preoperative (before drugs) patient and family
> Do preoperative patient assessment including family history, previous disease, lifestyle, and so forth to assist in planning home care
> Report outcomes to the nurse
>
> *Assignments*
> Develop a home plan of care for a specific type of surgical patient including resources needed and nutrition, and physical activity
> Present plan of care to a staff meeting

hand how nurses in the OR carry out their duties as patient advocates of persons who are worthy of recognition as individuals and not as procedures or inanimate objects. Perioperative nurses' caring acts of offering something as simple as a warm blanket, using touch to communicate reassurance, and assisting the patient to use personally effective coping mechanisms are all simple examples of the core values of respecting the dignity, worth, and humanness of each surgical patient.

LEVELED END-OF-PROGRAM OUTCOMES

Many schools of nursing have end-of-program outcomes by which they seek to ensure that students achieve defined values and skill sets as program end goals. Although these program outcomes vary widely within the 50 states, one that is often

> **Box 3**
> **Senior level outcomes communication**
>
> *Outcome*
> Incorporate therapeutic communication techniques with clients across all settings
>
> *Learning experiences*
> Review laboratory values
> Surgical site verification
> Cultural relevancy
> HIPPA
> Informed consent
>
> *Assignments*
> Report findings to anesthesiologist and surgeon
> Complete paper and report on cultural beliefs regarding surgery
> Report at postconference on how surgical site verification was completed and followed through to protect the patient

addressed is that of communication. The outcome of communication can be leveled when using the OR as a clinical site.

A common example of the communication outcome is that at the sophomore level (**Box 1**) the student is able to identify techniques of therapeutic communication. The student who is in a perioperative setting for a clinical rotation can follow the perioperative nurse as that professional explains to the patient what is going to happen in the OR, completes the preoperative assessment data set on the patient, and confirms that data set with the surgical team. The student may then report during postconference or complete a paper on the student's understanding of how the perioperative nurse applies therapeutic communication principles. Before the clinical experience, the student reviews and studies therapeutic communication.

At the junior level (**Box 2**), the student should begin to use therapeutic techniques in specific patient care situations. The student who is in a perioperative clinical site can teach postoperative home care to the patient undergoing ambulatory surgery. Before such teaching, the student must review hospital policies with the perioperative nurse. Each student must also prepare for teaching by understanding the surgical procedure

---

Box 4
Knowledge, skills, and values learned in circulator role

Knowledge acquired

Anatomy and physiology

Ethics (eg, cancer patient in which further surgery will not result in prolongation of life and ensuing discussion by surgeon)

Patient advocacy

Culture

Correct site surgery

Documentation

Patient safety

Skills acquired

Reflective, normative thinking: should have's, would have's, could have's

Assessment (hands on before every surgical procedure)

Critical thinking (how do I protect the patient, what should concern me based on the assessment)

Basic skills (Foley catheter, preparation, IVs, pulse oxygen, fluid and electrolytes, transporting a patient, communication)

Adaptability (eg, the case was cancelled, new one scheduled in its place)

Values

Accountability

Lifelong learning

Teamwork

Ethical decision making

Use of HIPPA rules

Professionalism

Individualism

the patient is to undergo, the expected nursing care, and the physician's home care orders. Students must also participate in assessment (ie, the collection of data regarding the history of the patient, medications used, and previous surgeries to plan the care needed at home). The perioperative nurse should question the student as to why findings are important, helping to hone critical thinking and problem-solving skills as they relate to discharge planning, patient education, and home care.

Senior level outcomes (**Box 3**) incorporate therapeutic communication techniques with clients across all settings. During the senior year, students in a perioperative rotation review laboratory values on the chart and report abnormal or unusual findings to the anesthesiologist and provider surgeon. This is an important step because most students remain hesitant to communicate with physicians. Seniors also engage in discharge teaching with the surgical patient and their family and the student also reports to the family on patient status during surgery.

With a clinical experience in perioperative patient care, the student can see the many different roles that a nurse plays in the perioperative setting. Often, students who lack OR clinical experience view the perioperative nurse as simply the one who assists the surgeon, but cannot envision the broader scope of perioperative nursing practice. Too often, such inexperienced students think of the perioperative nurse as merely stationed at the OR bed, handing instruments to the surgeon. In reality, perioperative nursing encompasses a wide range of activities, performed in a variety of settings. Perioperative nursing practice is based on scientific knowledge, an understanding of the necessity for certain techniques of care, and knowing when to initiate them.[4] **Boxes 4** and **5** were developed to assist in gaining an understanding of how

---

Box 5
Skills, knowledge, and values learned in scrub role

Skills

Asepsis

Maintaining a sterile field

How to do legal counts

Use of advanced technology

Communication

Assertiveness

Knowledge

Instrumentation

Anatomy and physiology

Working as a team member

Holding to the standards

Values

Accountability for one's own actions

Lifelong learning (required to attend one chapter meeting of the Association of Perioperative Registered Nurses or staff meeting in which education is scheduled)

Respect for others

Teamwork

Individualism professional behaviors

certain roles within the perioperative setting can help the student to grasp the much broader range of knowledge, skills, and values needed in perioperative nursing.

Boxes 1–5 describe potential learning in just two of the roles that perioperative nurses assume in practice. There are many more that the student can experience in the perioperative setting. During perioperative practice, the nurse accepts responsibility for practice through the use and observance of standards of care and recommended practices set forth by the Association of Perioperative Registered Nurses. The perioperative setting can serve as a high-caliber setting for the student nurse to learn the art and science of nursing. Through standards of practice, the perioperative nurse can lead the student into an evidenced-based practice that demonstrates a high accountability and responsibility for learning, caring, and clinical knowledge.

For the OR to work effectively as a clinical site, the same elements that are used in other clinical experiences are important. Faculty and staff must work together to ensure the best learning experience for the student. Faculty must inform perioperative educators or clinical staff of expected outcomes and work in concert to develop a plan of learning that enhances the experience for the student. Staff should be knowledgeable of the expectations of the experience and the educator must also be aware of the expectations of the staff.

ACKNOWLEDGMENTS

I recognize Julie Teague, RN, senior patient care facilitator in the operating room and St Vincent's Hospital, for being open minded and willing to try new methods of teaching. Without their partnership this clinical could not have been successful. I also thank Maryanne Rizzlo and the National League of Nursing for their interest in perioperative nursing.

REFERENCES

1. National League of Nursing (2005, Dec). Despite encouraging trends suggested by the NLN's comprehensive survey of all nursing programs, large numbers of qualified applicants continue to be turned down. Available at: http://www.nln.org/newsreleases/. Accessed January, 2006.
2. Wagner D, Kee C, Gray DP. A historical decline of educational perioperative clinical experiences. AORN J 1995;62(5):771–82.
3. Think tank on perioperative learning experiences in the nursing curriculum. Available at: http://www.nln.org/plublications/index.htm. Accessed March 16, 2005.
4. Rothrock J. Alexander's care of the patient in surgery. St. Louis (MO): Mosby; 2007.

Perioperative Nursing Observational Experience in an Associate Degree Program

Patricia Losito, RN, MSN, ANP

KEYWORDS

- ADN • Observations • Operating room • Nursing students
- Educational partnerships • Perioperative nurses

Erie Community College (ECC) depends on various settings for assigned student nurse observation experiences. It is important to try to expose students to as many opportunities and career choices as the community has to offer. Our students experience multiple learning opportunities through a variety of observational experiences that follow our philosophy and theoretical framework. The Department of Nursing at ECC functions within the framework of the philosophy of the college. Course and clinical content are developed according to certain beliefs about individuals, wellness, culture, community, environment, nursing, nursing education, the teaching–learning process, and nursing practice (**Box 1**).

Many of these beliefs can serve as organizing principles for a student's operating room (OR) observation experience. As an increasing emphasis is placed on a consumer-driven, community-based health care system, clinical sites, both hospital-based and settings within the community such as homes, schools, ambulatory settings, long-term care facilities, shelters, and community gathering places are used for clinical experiences. All classroom and clinical rotations are developed with end-of-program competencies in mind. As perioperative nurses consider the value of their practice setting as a clinical site, consideration of such competencies is helpful in discussions with members of the academic faculty. At ECC, nursing faculty expects that, at the conclusion of the nursing program, the nursing student will be able to:

Develop a commitment to the profession of nursing
Communicate verbally, nonverbally, in writing, or through information technology
Demonstrate assessment of clients' health status by collecting, analyzing, and synthesizing relevant data

Erie Community College, North Campus, 6205 Main Street, Williamsville, NY 14221, USA
E-mail address: losito@ecc.edu

Perioperative Nursing Clinics 4 (2009) 87–95
doi:10.1016/j.cpen.2009.02.003
1556-7931/09/$ – see front matter © 2009 Elsevier Inc. All rights reserved.

Box 1
Framework of beliefs for course and clinical content

Individual

Complex, dynamic social beings

Rational, capable of thinking, feeling, and using the problem-solving process

Influenced by culture and life experiences

Possess emotional, physical, social, spiritual, and intellectual capabilities and needs

Has an ability to learn, is motivated to succeed, and can learn to be self-directed

Is in constant interaction with the environment

Changes and grows in relation to development cycles and environmental factors

Has primary responsibility for health care decisions

Should be assisted by health care providers to make knowledge-based, informed decisions

Wellness

Life-long process on a continuum in which individuals experience a personal, dynamic, and ever-changing state

Influenced by heredity, developmental changes, environmental factors, and lifestyle choices

To promote, maintain, and reach an optimal level of wellness, individuals must constantly adapt to changes in the environment, and perceive themselves as having reached a state of wellness

Optimal use of available resources assists individuals in achieving the maximum potential for daily living

Culture

A set of traditions and practices that are passed down from one generation to another

Includes attitudes, values, beliefs, and practices unique to a particular group which affect an individual's perception of health and the health care delivery system

Important factor to consider when assessing the client and family

Gender role, language, impact of crisis events, values, beliefs, and traditions are considered when assessing cultural background

Conclusions based on cultural background require both critical-thinking and careful consideration

Nursing care must be individualized to meet cultural beliefs and practices

Community

Comprised of both formal and informal groups of people

Members interact to maintain open channels of communication and work to benefit all members.

A healthy community

    Possesses a high degree of community awareness and autonomy

    Identifies, analyzes, and organizes its resources to meet the needs of its groups

    Encourages its members to participate in the problem-solving process

Environment

Encompasses both an internal component, (those factors which are within the individual) and an external component (those factors which are outside of the individual)

Both components affect the individual, families, groups, and communities

Continuously changing; directly impacts on a sense of wellness

Effective use of resources requires a multidisciplinary team

Quantity, quality, and type of stimuli within the client's environment needs to be assessed to facilitate achievement of an optimal level of wellness

Environment can produce two types of stimuli:

    Insufficient stimuli (places the is individual at risk for sensory deprivation)

    Excessive stimuli (places the individual is at risk for sensory overload)

Nursing

Both an art and an applied science

    Art of nursing encompasses such concepts as caring behaviors, compassion, empathy, therapeutic communication, and client education

    Science of nursing reflects a broad base of knowledge drawn from the biologic, physical, psychological, and sociologic disciplines, and basic economic concepts and technological advances (reflect the recent and ongoing changes in the health care delivery system)

Unique function of nursing focuses on the promotion, maintenance and restoration of health; involves the ability to assess, plan, analyze, and evaluate comprehensive care

Requires engagement and collaboration with individual, family, and other members of the health care team

Nursing education framework

General education competencies in the arts and sciences

Body of nursing knowledge (develop competent and safe skills)

Development of critical-thinking skills (apply the nursing process)

Define, organize, analyze, and explain health care problems

Prioritize, intervene, and evaluate nursing actions

Grounded in collaborative relationships with faculty (student and the teacher are partners in learning)

Teaching–learning process

Flexible, interactive, and mutually goal-directed process

Teacher-facilitated and learner-motivated process

Requires multidimensional resources to promote student discovery in a climate of mutual respect and trust

Learner assumes responsibility for active learning and continuous self-evaluation

Learning is a lifelong process of assimilating theoretical knowledge, clinical skills, and professional values (continuation of nursing education in baccalaureate nursing program encouraged)

Learning does not proceed in the same manner and rate for all learners

Variety of instructional strategies enriches the learning process

Nursing practice

Grounded in the nursing process (considered the framework for nurses' accountability)

State Nurse Practice Act (outlines the scope of professional practice) and the criteria developed by the American Nurses Association as set forth in "Standards of Clinical Nursing Practice" provide guidelines for clinical practice

Theoretical knowledge and clinical application grounded in a strong legal, ethical, and moral base

Formulate clinical judgments through the performance of accurate assessments, and the analysis and integration of knowledge and information

Demonstrate caring interventions to assist clients in meeting their needs

Provide health education to clients to promote and maintain health and reduce risks

Work collaboratively with clients and other members of the health care team to achieve client and organizational outcomes

Manage client care through the efficient use of human, physical, financial, and technological resources[1]

CURRICULUM FRAMEWORK

The Department of Nursing philosophy incorporates beliefs regarding the individual, health, culture, community, environment, nursing, and nursing education as noted in **Box 1**. This philosophy becomes the organizing framework of the curriculum. The components of the organizing framework of the nursing curriculum are built on the work of Travis and Ryan's[2] Illness–Wellness Continuum, categories of human functioning, categories of health alterations, stages of maturity, and nursing practice roles as developed by the National League of Nursing Council of Associate Degree Nursing Competencies Task Force.[3]

In addressing the Illness–Wellness Continuum, the curriculum begins with assessment and health promotion activities directed toward the healthy individual, progressing to nursing care of clients in preservation of optimal health status, restoration of health status, and culminating with restoration of health in clients with acute or complex health problems.

The eight nursing practice roles of the Associate Degree Nurse are implemented throughout the curriculum. These roles come from the Educational Competencies for graduates of Associate Degree Nursing Programs developed by the National League for Nursing Council of Associate Degree Nursing Competencies Task Force.[3] These roles are systematically integrated on the clinical evaluation tool each semester throughout the nursing curriculum. They each present concrete opportunities when observed in perioperative practice settings.

Professional Behaviors

Professional behaviors within nursing practice are characterized by commitment to the profession of nursing. The graduate of an associate degree nursing program adheres to standards of professional practice, is accountable for her or his own actions and behaviors, and practices nursing within legal, ethical, and regulatory frameworks. Professional behaviors also include a concern for others, as demonstrated by caring, valuing the profession of nursing, and participating in ongoing professional development.

Communication

Communication in nursing is an interactive process through which there is an exchange of information that may occur verbally, nonverbally, in writing, or through information technology. Those who may be included in this process are the nurse, client, significant support persons, other members of the health care team, and community agencies. Effective communication demonstrates caring, compassion, and cultural awareness, and is directed toward promoting positive outcomes and establishing a trusting relationship. Therapeutic communication is an interactive verbal and nonverbal process between the nurse and client that assists the client to cope with change, develop more satisfying interpersonal relationships, and integrate new knowledge and skills.

Assessment

Assessment is the collection, analysis, and synthesis of relevant data for appraising the client's health status. Comprehensive assessment provides a holistic view of the client, which includes dimensions of physical, developmental, emotional, psychosocial, cultural, spiritual, and functional status. Assessment involves the orderly collection of information from multiple sources to establish a foundation for provision of nursing care, and includes identification of available resources to meet client needs. Initial assessment provides a baseline for future comparisons that can be made to individualize client care. Ongoing assessment and reassessment are required to meet the client's changing needs.

Clinical Decision-Making

Clinical decision-making encompasses the performance of accurate assessments, the use of multiple methods to assess information, and the analysis and integration of knowledge and information to formulate clinical judgments. Effective clinical decision-making results in finding solutions, individualizing care, and assuring the delivery of accurate, safe care that moves the client and support persons toward positive outcomes. Evidenced-based practice and the use of critical thinking provide the foundation for appropriate clinical decision-making.

Caring Interventions

Caring interventions are those nursing behaviors and actions that assist clients in meeting their needs. These interventions are based on a knowledge and understanding of the natural sciences, behavioral sciences, nursing theory, nursing research, and past nursing experiences. Caring is the "being with" and "doing for" that assists clients to achieve the desired results. Caring behaviors are nurturing, protective, compassionate, and person-centered. Caring creates an environment of hope and trust, where clients' choices related to cultural values, beliefs, and lifestyles are respected.

Teaching and Learning

Teaching and learning processes promote and maintain health and reduce risks, and are implemented in collaboration with the client, significant support persons, and other members of the health care team. Teaching encompasses the provision of health education to promote and facilitate informed decision-making, achieve positive outcomes, and support self-care activities. Integral components of the teaching process include the transmission of information, evaluation of the response to teaching, and modification of teaching based on identified responses. Learning involves the assimilation of information to expand knowledge and change behavior.

Collaboration

Collaboration is the shared planning, decision-making, problem solving, goal-setting, and assumption of responsibilities by those who work together cooperatively, with open professional communication. Collaboration occurs with the client, significant support persons, peers, other members of the health care team, and community agencies. The nurse participates in the team-approach to holistic, client-centered care across health care settings. The nurse functions as an advocate, liaison, coordinator, and colleague as participants work together to meet client needs and move the client toward positive outcomes. Collaboration requires consideration of client needs, priorities and preferences, available resources and services, shared accountability, and mutual respect.

Managing Care

Managing care is the efficient, effective use of human, physical, financial, and technological resources to meet client needs and support organizational outcomes. Effective management is accomplished through the processes of planning, organizing, directing, and controlling. The nurse, in collaboration with the health care team, uses these processes to assist the client to move toward positive outcomes in a cost-effective manner, to transition within and across health care settings, and to access resources.

Categories of human functioning include the following: protective (safety); sensory-perceptual (cognitive-perceptual); comfort, rest, activity, and mobility (activity, sleep and rest); nutrition (nutritional-metabolic); growth and development; fluid and gas transport; psychosocial-cultural functions (psychosocial dimensions); and elimination. Many of these have direct implications for learning in a perioperative practice setting, where an essential and elemental focus is on safety. This emphasis on safety embraces other categories of human function as the perioperative nurse considers sensory-perceptual alterations, problems with mobility, nutritional status, stages of growth and development, psychosocial status, and cultural needs in developing the plan of care.

Categories of health alterations include the immune, respiratory, cardiovascular, gastrointestinal, endocrine–metabolic, reproductive, integumentary–musculoskeletal, nervous–sensory, and renal–urinary systems along with psychosocial behaviors. These form the headings for the individual modules that comprise the theory and clinical courses. Alterations in any of the health systems and surgical intervention to correct or ameliorate the alteration are easily translated into part of the focus of a perioperative nursing observation.

The curriculum plan is designed so that coursework progresses in a logical and sequential pattern, from simple to complex, and from wellness to illness—encompassing the nursing process. The curriculum is presented to the students in a four-level approach. Critical thinking is demonstrated by each level's progression from knowledge at Level I to synthesis at Level IV. An emphasis on the application of critical thinking is incorporated in all courses. Each level builds on the content of the previous levels, including that of the sciences and humanities. Concepts of standard precautions and infection control are introduced in Level I and reinforced throughout the curriculum. Within each clinical course, the nurse's role in community-based settings is explored and examined.

Level I (first semester) deals with assessment and health promotion activities directed toward the healthy individual. Components include the theory courses Nursing (NU) 116 (Health Promotion) or NU 120 (Health Promotion: Registered Nurse Transition for Licensed Practical Nurse/Medical Military Personnel), and the clinical course NU 117. In addition, NU 128 (Physical Assessment), a nursing core corequisite for Level I, provides the knowledge base to enhance systematic assessment of clients throughout the life span and to evaluate clients along the wellness–illness continuum.

At Level II (second semester), the curriculum progresses to nursing care of clients in the preservation of optimal health status. The components include the theory course NU 126 (Health Maintenance) and the clinical course NU 127.

At Level III (third semester), the curriculum emphasizes the nursing care of clients in restoration of health status. The components include the theory course NU 236 (Health Restoration-Acute/Simple) and the clinical course NU 237.

Level IV (fourth semester) concludes the curriculum with the study of the restoration of health in clients with the focus on acute or complex health problems. The components include the theory course NU 246 (Health Restoration-Acute/Complex) and the clinical course NU 247. The nursing core corequisite for Level IV, NU 238 (Pharmacology for Nurses), provides students with knowledge of pharmacologic management for clients with commonly occurring alterations.

THE PERIOPERATIVE NURSING EXPERIENCE

Student's objectives for the perioperative observation experience are to describe the nurse's responsibilities for nursing care of the patient seeking health maintenance across the life cycle. Therefore, integrated into the perioperative nursing observation might be concepts such as fluid and electrolyte and acid–base imbalances, pain, and other concepts that characterize the perioperative experience for the patient undergoing an operative or other invasive procedure. The student uses the nursing process to interpret assessment data, select appropriate nursing diagnoses, and describe goals for health maintenance. After goal identification, students determine interventions for fluid and electrolyte and acid–base imbalances, pain management, and perioperative nursing care. They must also predict outcome measures that might be used to assess the effectiveness of care. The framework for the perioperative nursing observation follows the college's theoretical framework of an Illness–Wellness Continuum and can be related to the Perioperative Nursing Data Set (**Box 2**).[4] In every clinical assignment, including the one on perioperative nursing, the nursing student is required to address growth and development.

The nursing students are provided the opportunity to observe in the OR at multiple hospitals with which the college has clinical affiliating agreements. Students have the good fortune to attend a college in an area that has a level one adult trauma center, a pediatric hospital, and a cancer institute. The students are afforded this opportunity during the second semester of their freshman year. The perioperative setting affords numerous opportunities for our students to focus on acquisition of knowledge, skills, and values of importance to all nursing students (**Box 3**).

All of the clinical sites where a perioperative experience takes place have been responsive to our students and their learning needs. As in other parts of the country, we are competing for the same clinical sites with other colleges and universities.[5] The faculty has been instrumental in networking throughout the agencies by either past experiences or previous students that are now employed in these areas, to assure a positive experience. The communication between the facility and faculty has been the key component in these very brief but successful observations. Educational

---

Box 2
The perioperative nursing data set

Domains

Safety

Physiologic responses

Behavioral responses

Outcomes

Nursing interventions & activities

Outcome indicators

Box 3
Examples of student learning opportunities in perioperative practice settings

Knowledge

Anatomy, physiology, and pathophysiology

Ethical or legal responsibilities

Research applications

Safety concepts

Infection control

Teamwork

Resource use

Patients' or clients' diverse needs

Skills

Aseptic technique

Patient assessment

Communication

Organization

Coordination

Collaboration

Critical thinking

Decision-making

Assess interest and talent for perioperative practice

Values

Respect for human dignity

Right to self-determination

Protection of privacy

Maintainance of confidentiality

Advocacy

Multidisciplinary teamwork

Diverse career opportunities

Data from Baker, JD & Seifert, PC. Faculty Program, Part I-Using perioperative practice settings as clinical sites for nursing students. AORN 55th Congress, Wednesday, April 2, 2008.

---

partnerships, where clear goals are articulated, mutual expectations defined, and mutual planning undertaken have been described as one strategy to help alleviate the nursing faculty shortage.[6] In our partnerships, the contact person at the facility takes extreme care in matching the student with a patient undergoing surgery in an OR that embraces student learning and surgeons that enjoy teaching. The nursing students are to observe and report on the nursing role throughout the patient's progression from admission to discharge.

The verbal feedback from the staff has been positive. However, the staff and the students have expressed that the rotation should be longer. The students spend 1 day in the OR during their second semester. In addition, a recurring theme reported by the students is how amazed they are regarding the impact that perioperative nurses have on patients' total well being throughout the operative experience.

Throughout the nursing program, students are provided with multiple observations. The OR is unique in that, although it is a positive experience, the students report that they either they "love it" or "hate it"; there seems to be no middle ground. This type of response is quite evident when the students are evaluating their experience in the OR observation. As noted by Sigsby,[7] students who are attracted to perioperative nursing find it an exciting area of practice, where cutting edge technology prevails, and autonomy and camaraderie coexist on the OR team. These students express an ultimate goal of working in the OR. In the past, it was the requirement that new graduates have at least 1 year of medical or surgical experience. Recently, some hospitals have started to selectively hire new graduates for the OR. It is more vital than ever to continue to provide OR observation experiences for nursing students. These experiences could ultimately facilitate the potential opportunity for the new graduate nurse to achieve his or her goal of working in the OR.

For the nursing student who "loves" the OR observation, there is the opportunity to seek further exposure to the practice setting by seeking a nurse externship. As noted by Johnson,[8] nursing externships allow the student to "get the feel" for a particular practice area, perhaps find their niche in nursing, identify potential job prospects, and make themselves more marketable on graduation.

REFERENCES

1. Faculty at Erie Community College. Erie Community College nursing student handbook. Williamsville (NY); 2008. p. 5–8.
2. Travis JW, Ryan RS. Wellness workbook. Berkeley (CA): Ten Speed Press; 1988.
3. Faculty at Erie Community College. National League for Nursing. National league of nursing council of associate degree nursing competencies task force. New York; 2000.
4. Peterson C, editor. The perioperative nursing data set. 2nd edition [revised]. Denver (CO): AORN; 2007.
5. Lostio PM. Value of perioperative clinical learning activities in undergraduate nursing curricula. In: Losito PM, editor. Perioperative standards and recommended practices. Denver (CO): The Association; 2008.
6. Allan JD, Aldebron JD. A systematic assessment of strategies to address the nursing faculty shortage, U.S. Nurs Outlook 2008;50(6):286–96.
7. Sigsby LM. A voluntary summer program to expose nursing students to the perioperative specialty. AORN J 2008;88(4):609–17.
8. Johnson LA. Refine your clinical skills with a nursing externship. American Nursing Student 2008;10(1):1–3.

Simulation in Nursing Education

Janice A. Neil, RN, PhD

KEYWORDS

- Simulation • High fidelity • Perioperative
- Nursing education • Practice

SIMULATION IN NURSING EDUCATION

Clinical simulation is rapidly becoming important in nursing education as a viable supplement or substitute for practice with live patients. Although simulation can never replace actual clinical practice, it is a useful tool for creating realism before performing hands-on skills during patient care. Simulation can create realistic scenarios that not only test knowledge, but also provide a safe environment for practicing advanced concepts and difficult patient situations. Nursing faculty members are often challenged to prepare nurses for complex environments and work with interdisciplinary teams. In addition, health care administrators expect basic competence from new nursing graduates who are prepared to function in the complex work environment independently after orientation. Simulation may be the missing piece that can be added to a strong curriculum that is otherwise working well. Static manikins are useful for skill acquisition, but are often not adequate for learning or testing purposes. The new generation of nursing students is often video and computer savvy, and case studies and computer interactive CDs may not be as effective as possible with this new generation of learners.[1]

While simulation can be used in nursing education and hospital orientation programs, it can also be used to test basic competence, to practice rarely occurring emergency scenarios, and to assess readiness for clinical environments.[2] By definition, "A simulation resembles reality. In special reference to health care, simulation is an attempt to replicate some or nearly all of the essential aspects of a clinical situation so that the situation may be more readily understood and managed when it occurs for real in clinical practice."[3]

Simulations may be viewed as on a continuum from low-fidelity, including case studies and role play to partial task-trainers (intravenous [IV] cannulation arms or low-technology mannequins), to high-fidelity, sophisticated, computer-based simulations.[4] Simulation mimics reality and scenarios should be designed to not only test psychomotor competency, but also to assess critical thinking through role-play with

College of Nursing, East Carolina University, Greenville, NC 27858, USA
E-mail address: neilj@ecu.edu

Perioperative Nursing Clinics 4 (2009) 97–112
doi:10.1016/j.cpen.2009.02.002
1556-7931/09/$ – see front matter © 2009 Elsevier Inc. All rights reserved.

the use of sophisticated devices such as interactive videos and mannequins. Through simulation-based pedagogy, students can better integrate psychomotor, critical thinking, and communication skills to gain confidence before entering the clinical setting. Clinical simulation is rapidly earning a place in nursing education as a viable option to supplement clinical practice with live patients.

Simulation encourages active learning by engaging students. Students have different learning styles that can be incorporated into simulation scenarios. These include auditory, kinesthetic, visual, olfactory, and emotionally experiential learning styles.[2] Patient simulation provides students with experiences and skills that they might not obtain in clinical rotations. In addition, simulation can replace clinical rotations that have historically been observational.[5] Time can be suspended to allow students to think critically, to make decisions, and to act without the pressure of a fast-paced hospital environment where students may not have a clear picture or be prepared to act in timely fashion. For many years, nursing programs have used laboratories to simulate patient situations using static mannequins, supplies, and equipment.

Today, however, computerized human simulators, accompanied by sophisticated scenarios, can create high-level clinical situations.[5] Some of the concepts that can be reinforced with computerized simulation are patient safety, resuscitation, and clinical judgment. The key concepts of the class can be used to develop simulations. In fact, some schools of nursing substitute simulation for clinical experiences because of lack of access to hospitals and clinical sites. Recognizing this access issue, the State Board of Nursing of California states that up to 25% of clinical rotations may take place in simulation situations although the simulations must include actual demonstrations that encompass the nursing process.[2]

Simulation appeals to technology-savvy students to whom lecture, passive information, and linear thinking may not provide full engagement. Today's students have been immersed in technology from an early age and they learn differently. Simulation is a more comfortable medium for students to coordinate cognitive, affective, and psychomotor skills. As simulation becomes a more popular mode of teaching in nursing programs, new graduates coming to the perioperative area with be increasingly familiar with it and can adapt easily to simulations related to being a perioperative nurse.[6]

Motivating students often involves active participation, individualized instruction, and prompt feedback. Simulation can help to attain key goals in nursing education such as critical thinking, decision making, interactive learning, confidence building, remediation or reinforced learning, and crossing the bridge between practicum and classroom.[7] Learners need to apply knowledge for the scenario to be effective. All simulations should include a debriefing session where a videotape of the simulation is shown and the critique of performance can occur. Constructive feedback is important at this time. Instructors and peers need guidelines in the debriefing process so that no one feels inferior or inept.

Implementation of simulation depends on the level of the students. The novice user should begin with low- or medium-fidelity simulators and scenarios. These might include learning basic nursing skills and performing physical assessment. The intermediate student can be moved to patient scenarios with higher fidelity that involve complex procedures and concepts frequently occurring in nursing. The advanced user can then be moved to high-fidelity simulations with complex interwoven concepts and skills. It is advisable to begin with lower fidelity simulation or a thorough orientation to simulation before using high-fidelity simulation for the first time. Not being oriented to the room, the simulator itself, or the process can cause a scenario to go awry and allow ineffective teaching to result.[2]

BRIEF HISTORY OF SIMULATION

Simulation is not unique to medicine or nursing. Simulation has been used for many years in many industries. **Table 1** provides examples of several types of simulators.

Simulation first arose within the aviation industry. In the earliest days of flight, pilots realized that training was required before taking the controls of even "simple" aircraft.[10] Simulation began in the late 1920s to train pilots in the skill of "blind" or instrument flying.[11] The first device, the Sanders Teacher, was a mock aircraft that was mounted on the ground facing the wind. The Link Trainers were a series of ground simulators created between the 1930s and early 1950s. These were developed to train pilots to fly using instrument flight rules.[10] Computers were added to flight simulators in the 1940s. NASA and the space program contributed to advances in simulation by adding digital computers to improve the capabilities of flight simulators. Today, modern commercial flight simulators provide realistic full control replication and motion bases or platforms to provide cues of real motion.[10]

Patient simulators have been used in nursing for more than 50 years.[12] The first simulations in nursing were performed with "Resusci Anne and Harvey" in the 1960s.[4] Åsmund S. Lærdal began the development of a realistic and effective training aid to teach mouth-to-mouth resuscitation using a model of an unidentified woman for his new resuscitation-training manikin, Resusci Anne. The original "Anne" was said to duplicate a woman pulled out of the River Seine in Paris in 1900 who was never identified. Lærdal was convinced that if a manikin were life-sized and life-like, students would be better motivated to learn resuscitation techniques. Also in the 1960s, prehospital emergency medicine began to be seen as an extension of advanced hospital treatment. Portable training aids soon developed to simulate ventilation and airway control. In the 1980s, anesthesia educators studied how simulation was being used in aviation and military training, and began using simulation in the anesthesia-training environment.[13]

The widespread use of simulators blossomed in the 1990s.[12] Technical skills such as airway management, vascular catheter insertion and vaginal delivery were first practiced with task-training models.[12] Nurse anesthesia faculty and students were the first to use high-fidelity simulation and it has now expanded to include critical care, acute care, perioperative, and emergency nursing.[12] In 2000, Laerdal produced

Table 1
Examples of different types of simulation and their historical purpose

Type	Purpose
Virtual	Using virtual equipment and real people[8]
Aircraft	Pilot training[8]
Virtual body	Training in medicine[8]
Nuclear reactor/power plant	Reactor operation and disposal of used nuclear fuel[8]
Construction/earthquake	Design of buildings and bridges that can withstand earthquakes[8]
Business	Predictive displays, policy, conflict management[8]
Virtual ship	Ship building and navigation[8]
Fire and police departments	Controlled fires, negotiating, disasters[4]
Motor vehicle companies	"Crash-dummies"[4]
Models of Population Dynamics	Explore future burdens of chronic disease by health policy makers[9]

SimMan, the high-fidelity simulator.[4] Since then, Laerdal and other companies have developed several high-fidelity mannequins in use today.

THE TECHNOLOGY OF SIMULATION
Types of Simulation

The nurse educator must understand the different types and levels of simulation. The word "simulation" should be used with caution because it is a broad term that incorporates many types and levels. The type of simulation selected necessarily reflects the objectives of the teaching and learning session.

The types and levels of medical and nursing simulation may be classified as follows[2]:

Low fidelity: includes disembodied body parts for specific skill performance. These are often "task-trainers." Examples include IV arms and pelvic models for Foley catheter insertion.

Computer assisted instruction: live interactions with a simulated patient that may include preprogrammed decisions about care and the result. Examples are Sim-Hosp, SimClinic, and VirtualIV. Another tool has three-dimensional visualization that allows ways to study anatomy. In addition, there are many web-based technologies developed for nursing instruction that are bundled with textbooks, workbooks, or software packages.

Moderate fidelity: provide some feedback to students. Usually these mannequins can produce sounds that can be used for evaluative purposes. An example is Vital-Sim (Laerdal/Medical).[2] Some task-trainers fall into this category, such as equipment used to learn robotic and laparoscopic surgery techniques.

High fidelity: this type of simulator is the most complex and includes computerized components that can be programmed to produce lifelike scenarios and which react to student's manipulations in realistic ways by speaking and coughing. Mannequins display chest and eye movement, and respond to pharmacologic interventions and physical manipulations. The operator programs simulations or operates the mannequin manually via a computer linked to the mannequin. Some examples are SimMan (Laerdal/Medical), iStan (METI) and Hal (Gaumard Scientific).

A high-fidelity simulator may include a cardiovascular system with palpable pulses, heart sounds, measurable blood pressure, EKG waveforms, and invasive parameters such as arterial, central venous, and pulmonary artery pressures. Respiratory components may include regulated spontaneous ventilations, measurable exhaled gasses, and audible breath sounds. Other parts of such a simulator may include a pharmacologic system that responds to anesthetic, analgesic, and vasoactive agents and a urological system that can be filled to simulate urine output. In some high-fidelity mannequins, the pupils are reactive. Defibrillation, needle cricothyroidotomy, jet ventilation, needle thoracentesis, and chest tube insertion can also be performed.[12]

The METI (Sarasota, FL) high-fidelity simulators have four components. They include a mannequin, a freestanding enclosure with simulation components, a computer to integrate the functions of the simulator components, and an interface that allows users to control the simulation and modify physiologic parameters.[14] Once the operator loads a prewritten scenario, the program runs and responds to modifications.[12]

There are many advantages and challenges associated with simulation. These are outlined in **Table 2**. Simulation has many advantages, not least of which is to allow students to develop critical thinking skills and to analyze their own actions. Students

Table 2	
Advantages and challenges of simulatione	
Advantages	**Challenges**
Allows student to critically analyze their actions and to reflect on their skill sets.[4]	Expense: start-up. equipment, and maintenance.[4,12,15]
Ability to critique the performance of others and compare it to themselves.[4]	Troubleshooting and operation.[4]
Students are allowed to make errors and can learn from them in a safe environment.[4]	Space needed for multiple components.[4]
The instructor does not have to "take over" as often happens in the clinical area when patient safety is at risk.[4]	Advancing computer literacy skills.[4,15]
Decreased levels of performance anxiety and heightened sense of self-confidence in psychomotor and critical thinking skills can develop.[13,15]	Available technical support: at least two people are needed for a simulation, the operator and the person guiding the simulation.[12]
Uncommon critical and clinical problems can be simulated.[12]	A tendency to create hypervigilance or exaggerated caution.[12]
Allows standardized testing and management of errors[12] and real-time feedback[15]	Extensive faculty commitment and support; faculty must be trained in scenario writing.[12]
Actively involving learners.[12]	Overgeneralizations can occur that do not mimic real-world scenarios.[12]
Providing relatively consistent experiences for all students.[12]	Anatomic models despite their many capabilities are not human. There can be incomplete presentation of reality.[12]
Collecting physiologic, video, and audio data for reflective sessions.[12]	Transfer of learning from a simulated environment to clinical practice has not been well researched and documented.[12]
Real patient care on simulated patient.[16]	Financial constraints related to purchase of expensive equipment.[15]
Focused training; team training.[15,16]	Possible need for renovation to accommodate technologies.[15]
Dedicated space for training.[16]	Added computer literacy.[15]
"Suspension of disbelief": realistic scenarios, realistic equipment, realistic patient conditions.[15,16]	Curricular changes needed to incorporate simulation.[15]
Avoidance of negative training and transfer; ability to identify results and outcomes related to interventions.[16]	Need for a focused pedagogy and vision for simulation.[15]
Decreased student anxiety and increased self-confidence for students learning new skills.[15]	Naysayers and pessimists are in many faculty groups.[5]
Potentially less stress than live clinical activities.[15]	
Shorter orientation programs at health care facilities for new graduates and new nurses.[15]	
Improved clinical performance and competency.[15]	
Less stress than live clinical activities.[15]	
Enhanced critical thinking.[15]	
Increased opportunities for practice.[15]	

are also able to critique the performance of others, and they can make errors without the instructor having to step in for patient-safety reasons. This enables better learning, allowing students to see the gravity of errors that they might have made. Often following simulation, there is decreased performance anxiety in clinical settings because students have been able to practice in supportive, less stressful environments. Simulation also allows for standardized testing and experience with infrequently occurring events. Above all, simulation includes active learning and doing, team training, increased opportunities for practice, and enhanced critical thinking.

There are also many challenges associated with simulation. Simulation can be expensive and time consuming. It requires large expenditures of capital and often needs troubleshooting. For high-fidelity simulation, a trained operator and faculty who are committed and computer savvy must be present. Some report a hypervigilance with students that may not be present in the clinical area. Anatomic models, despite their many simulated capabilities, are not human. There can be incomplete presentation of reality. Overgeneralizations can occur that do not always mimic real-world scenarios. Finally, the curriculum may need to be changed to reflect focused pedagogy and a vision for simulation.

Getting Started with Simulation

Funding is often the first consideration because simulators may cost $50,000 to $250,000 each. Additional programs for the simulator may add $30,000. The cost of disposable goods including IV fluids, tubing, dressing supplies, and props must also be considered.[5]

In order for expensive high-fidelity simulation to be used effectively, several preliminary steps must occur. Faculty support is the key to integrating simulation into the curriculum.[5] The faculty members must see the value in simulation and become familiar with running the simulator, preparing students for the scenario.[5] Some institutions allow release time for faculty members to become oriented to the simulator and for training and writing scenarios. However, many prewritten scenarios are available though the vendors. When writing or purchasing scenarios, faculty must keep in mind that the student experience depends on the reality of the scenarios and the presentation. The instructor must be able to engage the students in the care of the patient while the situation progresses or is suspended while students make decisions. The scenario should prompt students to perform all the skills that they normally would at a health care facility.

There are always obstacles. Naysayers and pessimists are in many faculty groups.[5] Those eager to learn and experience simulator should be the focus of the proponent administrators.

The faculty and operators will need to attend seminars for simulation training. When a simulator arrives at a facility, the faculty is faced with a life-sized mannequin that has a compressor, a power control unit, and a laptop. The newest simulators can blink, speak, and breathe. They have a simulated heartbeat and a pulse. The simulators can respond physiologically with bradycardia, hypotension, or even death. A slave screen is also included so heart rhythm, waveforms, and invasive monitor readings can be viewed.

Accordingly, the faculty requires orientation to this sophisticated piece of equipment and usually a multiple-day workshop by the vendor is included for those who will be operating the simulator. The workshop focuses on the science of simulation and basic simulator operation. Included in these vendor seminars are the educational concepts surrounding simulation, writing scenarios, and operation of the computerized components.[6] Part of the training must be hands-on so that instructors can learn to manipulate the computer program and witness the myriad possible changes in the human patient simulator.[5]

When faculty start to use the simulator, it is advisable to start at a simple level and move to ever more complex levels as students advance through the program. Simulation scenarios should be developed using the course objectives, the nursing process, decision making, and discussion of student reactions.[6] In addition, National Council Licensure Examination testing areas and score reports can be used to identify strengths and weaknesses in a program where simulation might be useful. Credibility is enhanced by using these test plan categories. Communication with clinical facilities about recent graduates may also help to identify areas where scenarios can be developed and implemented.

From there, it is important to decide what type of data collection is desired from the simulation scenarios and how it will be used. Faculty who are involved in the implementation process and who assist with simulation development will be more likely to embrace the technology.[15] Some institutions create simulation committees. Such committees often review templates for content, accuracy, current evidenced-based practice, and unnecessary distractions.[15]

There are several ways to run scenarios. They include an "on the fly" or as you go, an ad hoc approach. This allows maximum flexibility, requires no prewritten program, and has minimal upfront time investment. However, this type of operation requires an attentive, dynamic instructor with content knowledge who is able to respond quickly to student interventions.

Another type is the automatic, preprogrammed style. This is more rigid and requires significant upfront time investment. In addition, it requires an operator with knowledge of the software who can preprogram the computer that will run the simulator. In these preprogrammed simulations, the simulator (mannequin) responds to student interventions. These scenarios can be standardized for evaluation and research. Once developed, these scenarios can be part of the curriculum.[15]

Any simulation scenario must have a design template that includes the "patient" data and history, psychomotor and cognitive skills required before simulation, the setting and environment, and the type of simulator manikin needed. Significant lab values, physician orders, and student information are needed before running the scenario. Props and equipment that are needed should be listed and be available in the room. This also includes medications, IV fluids, and documentation forms. Each scenario should include the recommended mode for simulation, and roles and guidelines for the roles.[15] Errors should also be imbedded so that critical thinking and problem solving can occur. The simulation should be set up and ready to go when the participants enter the room.[17]

Student preparation should begin as early in the education program as possible. Each student should receive a comprehensive orientation about the simulation center. Before each simulation, another brief orientation should occur that includes available supplies and medications. In addition, before the simulation, students should be given reading assignments, guidelines on participating in the simulation, standard simulation objectives, and the patient's case summary (**Box 1**).[17,18] Instructor training should be uniform. If there is more than one instructor, minimal variability exists so that students receive consistent learning experiences. Support for instructors should include a person who is very familiar with simulation. A clear articulation of roles is helpful in providing consistency among faculty members.[17] In addition, each actor needs specific guidelines regarding his or her role and recommended responses to student inquiries. Often the actor playing the patient's voice only gives information that the student requests.[17]

> **Box 1**
> **Information that should be provided to students before a simulation**
>
> Patient "report" and physical condition
>
> Admission and current status
>
> Monitoring devices
>
> Treatment
>
> Psychosocial information and issues
>
> *Data from* Lamond D, Crow R, Chase J, Doggen K, Swinkels M. Information sources used in decision making: Considerations for simulation development. Int J Nurs Stud. 1996;33(1):47–57.

The final component of simulation is the reflective discussion or debriefing session. This is the most critical component of the learning experience. Debriefing allows the instructors to review specific student behaviors and decision making related to the scenario objectives. This process should allow students to evaluate themselves and their peers. Student successes should be discussed first. Faculty should focus on key issues that are defined by the objectives. If grading is part of the simulation, points are often awarded for each completed task.[17]

Following are other important concepts relative to nursing practice where simulation can be used.

HEALTH PROMOTION

Health promotion has long been an important aspect of nursing practice. Simulation can be used by health planners for prevention programs using models to explore the future burden of chronic diseases. These models can convey the structure of inflow of adult population growth related to certain diseases that is grounded in the scientific literature. Jones and colleagues[9] created a model to describe the dynamics of diabetes related to populations. Included in this model were US Census Bureau data, the National Health and Interview Survey, the National Health and Nutrition Examination Survey, the Behavioral Risk Factor Surveillance System, and the research literature. The US Census Bureau data includes population growth and death rates and health insurance coverage. The National Health Interview Survey reports disease prevalence and detection. The National Health and Nutrition Examination Survey reports prechronic condition prevalence (such as prediabetes), and the Behavioral Risk Factor Surveillance System reports monitoring efforts and physical examination data. The purpose of this simulation modeling was not only prediction, but also possible prevention strategies that could be used to change the future of chronic disease.[9]

SAFETY

Safety in the health care arena has been in the forefront following the Institute of Medicine's report on improved patient safety.[19] The use of simulation was fueled, in part, by the Institute of Medicine's report on improved patient safety. There is now a heightened awareness of patient safety issues in the clinical settings and the prevention of untoward events. Simulation can assist with this by providing safe environments to practice safety issues.[17] The case study approach can be a guideline for simulation. Using case studies as a guide, simulation has the advantages of improving student abilities to meet course objectives around safety concepts. Using simulation demands careful attention to the details of the simulation, debriefing, and evaluation process. There must be clear, measurable objectives. Case studies and computer simulations often lack the essential elements of enabling students to interact with patients and family members, and settings that mimic the actual care environment. High-fidelity simulation can bridge the gap between theory and practice by allowing students to practice skills in realistic situations without potentially harming patients, thus enhancing safety concepts. In addition, safety issues or untoward events at a facility can be reviewed using simulation in an effort to educate and evaluate safety risks. Part of the growing interest in simulation stems from the increased interest in patient safety. The old adage, "see one, do one, teach one," that has often been the accepted method for developing expertise has been replaced by "see one, practice many, do one, and teach one by using simulation methods."[20]

The debriefing process around safety issues has a main goal to promote student self-assessment and learning for increasing critical thinking skills. Stressing that mistakes are part of the learning process and it is much better to make an error with a simulator than with an actual patient, especially surrounding safety issues, is paramount. Analysis of the thinking process that often leads to the errors can also be discussed. Student feelings can be validated and simulation allows students to confront uncomfortable feelings and deal with them in a controlled and safe setting versus a clinical setting. The debriefing format requires that a set amount of minutes occur after the simulation to review feelings and questions while they are fresh in the student's mind. If the scenario is graded, students can be given their simulation videos, debriefing questions, and points awarded. In some cases, a second debriefing session may occur once students have time to reflect on their experiences.[20]

ETHICAL CONSIDERATIONS

There are areas of growing importance related to simulation that will need to be addressed as the popularity of simulation in nursing education progresses. One area regards the ethical implications that include professional implications, and desirable research and development. "Simulation is a goal oriented experimentation using dynamic models; those with time-dependent behavior".[8] It provides application areas related to alternative courses of action, acquisition of knowledge, prototyping, diagnosis, testing concepts, and understanding.[8] The issues of patient safety and the challenge to promote student learning and competency through increased use of simulations requires nurse educators to consider the ethical considerations of integrating simulation as an education strategy in the teaching, learning, and evaluative processes.[4] Questions arise about social justice; should students be prepared and competencies validated through simulation before providing patient care?[4] Is simulation a reliable method to evaluate student competence? Since high-fidelity simulation is a new entity in nursing programs, and not yet embraced by all, will students in the future be required to demonstrate competence before giving patient care? In other words, as simulation becomes more popular and more sophisticated, will first-time procedures on actual patients not be allowed? The principles of autonomy, beneficence, nonmaleficence, veracity, and compassion all can be argued as reasons to require simulation before actual patient experiences. However, these conflict with several norms that currently exist in nursing education; nursing students "practice" on live patients. The professional implications fall into three concepts: knowledge, activity. and behavior. Knowledge is necessary as a beginning step that yields the activities for acceptable behavior. Ethical implications include the proper guidelines to guide simulation. Certification for simulationists has been proposed as an important step in the maturity of simulation.[8]

Currently in some institutions, real "patients" are used as simulated patients as a way of collecting data. These trained and coached real-life patients are told to behave or act in a certain manner. In addition, they are given a list of symptoms to present to the person practicing or being tested. Controversy exists about deceiving a professional about the true reason for a visit; in some cases, students are tricked into thinking that the person is a real patient instead of an actor.[21] The use of real people in simulations can be useful for direct observation and interviewing, but deception should not occur. High-fidelity simulation has the potential to eliminate real "patient" actors and can be just as effective as a pedagogic tool.

CRITICAL THINKING

Critical thinking is often difficult to teach because it is an abstract concept. In addition, there are no standard models of exactly what critical thinking is. Computer-based and high-fidelity simulation can be used as a method to teach students content and critical thinking skills without using actual live patients. Nursing educators know the importance of critical thinking skills. These skills can be enhanced in instructional methods that stimulate critical thinking. Many instructors feel that giving students a variety of clinical experiences would enhance critical thinking skills. However, this is often not the case because more variety often leads to observation experiences where little or no critical thinking occurs. More controlled critical thinking exercises are helpful in building skills where the student participates in the exercise. Simulation can be an effective method of teaching critical thinking skills safely and independently of the instructor.[22]

A meta-analysis of nine quantitative studies related to simulation by Ravert revealed that 75% of the studies showed positive effects of simulation on skill and knowledge acquisition.[23] However, more research is needed on high fidelity simulation and its effect on critical thinking in nursing education. One of the main weaknesses is the uncertain reliability and validity of current evaluative instruments. So far, limited research exists to validate the effectiveness of simulation in building critical thinking skills.[23] However, the advantages noted in the literature include the ease of presenting serious and uncommon situations, self-paced learning, developing higher order thinking skills, and students erring without repercussions to learner or patient. In addition, there is the potential for immediate feedback and reinforcement that can be applied consistently across learners.[23]

Reported disadvantages of simulation include lack of realism in the simulation experience and the expense of high-fidelity, computer-based simulators.[23] Educators are charged with educating and ensuring competence and static simulations are often part of the process. High-fidelity simulations are a recent addition to health care education, but research is needed to investigate the best ways to use high-fidelity simulation for maximum benefit. In addition, evidenced-based practice can be introduced and simulated.

Examples of Simulation Used in Undergraduate Nursing Education

The literature contains reports of many specialized types of simulation projects. Simulation is an evolving art and it is not always a preferred method of learning by students. Some examples of specialized simulation projects are noted below.

Parr and Sweeney[5] used simulation in an acute coronary syndrome and myocardial infarction scenario for senior nursing students in a critical care course.[5] This involved five students working as a team and two critical care faculty members, one running the simulator. Students needed to prepare ahead of time. Before simulation, students were given a synopsis that included history, emergency department orders, and a list of study questions. Students were then introduced to the simulator by name. They were to assess the patient, pick up key findings in his assessment and history, and plan his care. Soon the patient moved into cardiogenic shock with chest pain, worsening hypotension, decreased oxygen saturation, and premature ventricular contractions. The students used the standing orders to determine what medications to administer. A great deal of time was spent calculating a medication bolus and infusion. Finally, the patient was transferred to the cardiac catheterization lab for angioplasty and stent placement.[5]

One of the most essential skills needed by every nurse is IV catheter insertion. In most schools of nursing, instruction is provided in clinical laboratories with static task-trainer simulators. More sophisticated computerized simulators consist of models of "patient" arms with graphics of veins, skin, and musculature. Nursing educators have scarce evidence about best practices in employing these new technologies to facilitate student learning. Woody and Cherry[24] completed a study where students had to be engaged in critical thinking to determine why the patient needed an IV access and what type of access would be most appropriate for that patient. Each student had to select which site to explore for IV insertion and determine which vein would offer the best access for the catheter size chosen. The student then gathered all supplies and proceeded with the steps to insert the IV catheter. The purpose of the study was to explore students' perceptions of learning IV skills in the clinical laboratory setting, and whether they preferred the computerized simulator to static mannequin arms. Forty-four percent of the students felt that the simulator helped them to learn the steps in the procedure for starting an IV, but 55% of the respondents listed technical problems with the simulator and were frustrated.[24]

Roberson and colleagues'[25] study involved wound management and care. Wound care is often a challenge for students. Malodorous wounds are a common problem. The sense of smell plays a vital role in our sense of well-being and quality of life. It also serves as a recognition function and assessment tool. Their study provided a multisensorial, high-fidelity simulation for wound care that incorporated olfactory elements to test a new method of simulation, and allowed students to develop coping strategies for dealing with malodorous wounds. The responses in the experimental group were significantly different ($P<.001$ in most cases) from the control group in 8 of 12 survey items indicating the addition of odor was beneficial in enhancing the perceived realism and value of the simulation. Furthermore, responses to open-ended questions suggested the addition of odor in the simulation laboratory improved realism and provided a safe environment for reacting to a wound. Finally, participants expressed high levels of confidence with their wound care skills after the study.

"Failure to rescue" is a term applied to clinical issues that are improperly treated and that lead to adverse outcomes. Young and colleagues[26] developed 12 scenarios to test medical students' and residents' reactions to basic floor emergencies. All groups had significant deficits in cognitive performance in the areas of evaluation, follow-up with presenting problems, and total performance. It was troubling for the researchers because often physicians are left to independently diagnose and intervene in life-threatening emergencies. A problem recognized was the difficulty in proving that simulated learning improves the efficiency and performance of trainees. Standardization of vignettes and grading are often necessary for accurate evaluation. There are quantitative and qualitative differences in decision making of novice clinicians in critical care simulations. Deliberate practice is essential to gaining effective experience. This includes using the mental processes that are needed for real-life situations. Simulation does not have to be high fidelity in nature to be effective. Active participation is the key element. Parts of a simulation such as a psychomotor task like tracheotomy care can be first separated from the main scenario in a task–trainer type device. When students are proficient in the task, an entire simulation that includes the task can then be incorporated. If students are uncomfortable with a procedure and it is part of the simulation, it can lead to anxiety, frustration, and simulations that go wrong. Therefore, task training may have to occur before scenarios are done.[27]

Uses of Simulation in the Orientation and Training of Perioperative Nurses

Mentoring for students and newly graduated perioperative nurses has long been the cornerstone of orientation programs. However, 69% of new nurses leave their place of employment within the first year.[28] The operating room is often an area where new nurse turnover rates are high. At a program in a hospital in the Midwest, only 44% of the new nurses continued to work as staff nurses for a year.[28] The student or new perioperative nurse must learn a great deal of new material in a technically complex work environment. New graduates are coming to the perioperative setting in larger numbers and they may feel isolated and discouraged. The Associate of Peri-Operative Registered Nurses' "Perioperative Nursing Course 101" is often a part of the orientation process for new nurses entering the perioperative area. This program is an excellent exposure to the operating room, but it may not help with satisfaction related to didactic and clinical areas. Most successful mentorship programs are built through personal interactions that add up over time. A mentorship program that includes simulation experiences may increase retention rates because new nurses will not have to experience new concepts and procedures with real patients in a highly charged operating room environment.[28]

One of the biggest challenges for students or new nurses working in the perioperative environment is communication. At a hospital in Michigan, there is a center with two mock operating rooms to allow surgical team members to rehearse interactions that can improve communication and patient care. One room is used to provide simulations on emergencies without the risk to an actual patient such as cardiac arrest, power outages, and fire in the operating room. The second room has task-trainers such as the da Vinci robot, and any new specialty equipment. Ten workstations are available to learn procedures ranging from suturing to complex surgical procedures for surgical residents. In addition, nursing staff can familiarize themselves with new equipment before actual use on patients. Procedures and objectives for both rooms are clear. The major concept for both rooms is patient safety.[29]

Simulation can be an effective method of teaching and learning for all perioperative staff. The best type of simulation is one where many types of professionals are involved and that can mimic a possible emergency where many people are involved. Scenarios are multidisciplinary to allow teams to develop strategies for dealing with seldom seen emergencies such as malignant hyperthermia. Dealing with these types of emergencies can also help student develop critical thinking skills in a more supportive environment, which could lead more students into perioperative nursing. The keys to effective simulation in the perioperative area include the following steps[30]:

1. Identify the target audience. This might include physicians, nurses, surgical technicians, pharmacists, and secretaries.[30] Participants should start with level 1 cases, and get more complex as they become familiar with simulation.[28]

2. Define clear objectives: examine past events or events that must be orchestrated quickly and effectively for good patient outcomes. Keep in mind the learning needs of the individuals in the room with open-ended questions and then form behavioral objectives with measurable outcomes for each group or person.

3. Develop relevant scenarios: include frequently occurring events and normal and abnormal events that occur in the perioperative area. The teamwork needed around life-threatening emergencies is a good type of scenario for teams. This also can expose a student to perioperative events that they might not see in their practicum. Scenarios can be simple or complex, but should not last any longer than 20 minutes. Usually some critical thinking and psychomotor components should be incorporated. Be sure to have some components that a student knows or can be involved in.

4. Determine assumptions and limitations: examine past events or knowledge to be tested. The leader must know the educational level of the people participating in the simulation. If people participating in the scenario are new to the perioperative setting, they should still have enough knowledge to participate the scenario. No one should feel humiliated because he or she cannot perform because of lack of training or knowledge. Prepare a detailed protocol, including:

   The title
   The concepts
   The length of the scenario
   The location
   The target population
   The learning objectives
   The roles need to carry out the scenario
   The scenario stem

5. Determine the fidelity level needed; there is no need to use high fidelity if the scenario can be played out on a low-fidelity simulator. It is important that if a high-fidelity simulator is used that the operator is trained in its use so that suspended reality can occur. The more realistic the scenario, the better the players will be able to carry out the scenario in a realistic way.

6. Determine the means of evaluation. Often scenarios are videotaped, so there should be a way to evaluate the scenario in the debriefing process. Standard guidelines are available, and Likert scales and checklists for evaluation. It is best that the person evaluating the simulation is not the same person operating the high-fidelity simulator.

7. Perform the simulation: The participants should also be oriented to simulation in general and the particular simulator that will be used. If the simulation is going poorly, the leader should intervene to put the participants back on track or stop the scenario altogether. There is no need to continue a scenario if things are going awry or the participants are confused and cannot perform.

8. Debrief the participants. The group should watch the videotape. Then each person can comment on the scenario. Avoid negativity and lead the debriefing using behavioral terms that were measurable.

Several large multidisciplinary simulation centers exist. At the Peter M. Winter Institute for Simulation Education and Research at the University of Pittsburgh, multidisciplinary training and research coexist. Their training programs use simulation-based education to provide a safer environment for patients of the University of Pittsburgh Medical Center and its affiliates.[31] At the University of Texas at Arlington, a "Smart Hospital and Health System" was developed. This is a 13-bed center where students interact with and provide care to a full array of patients in the "emergency room, labor and delivery, and ICU." Many levels of simulation are used.[32]

Another method of simulation aims at complex task training. In the laparoscopic world, everything is backward. Looking at the right translates into steering to the left. The longer the procedure takes, the higher the risk of complications for the patient. A reality-based trainer can help students learn how to manipulate the camera. Virtual reality-based training improves the operative performance of novices and seasoned professionals. For students, it allows them to become familiar with the type of equipment they might see in their rotation and how it works. Currently, only 55% of general surgery programs have a simulation skills lab. Since good surgical outcomes are critical and dependent on the entire team, simulation can be an important training tool.[33] Traditional surgical training has been performed on cadavers and animals, or on humans under the guidance of an attending physician. However, simulators allow users to repeat training sessions repeatedly, monitor progress, and maintain competency. Ethical issues related to using animals and the difficulty in procuring and preserving cadavers make simulation a viable alternative despite its initial start-up costs that can be as high as a million dollars. As simulation progresses and gains acceptance, honing skills during live procedures may no longer be acceptable. In addition, credentialing will become easier.[8,31]

Examples of operating room simulations that are useful for students include[34]:

Putting on surgical attire
Describing the general purpose and nature of surgery
Identifying and performing the roles of the circulating nurse
Setting priorities
Basic principles of surgical asepsis
Assisting with anesthesia
Safety precautions
Transferring and positioning
Time out
Patient identification
Environmental control
Traffic and stress
Record keeping
Emergencies
Operating room readiness.

For the postanesthesia-care unit, some of the possible simulations include:

Parameters for assessment of new patients
Cardiac rhythm anomalies
Post-operative bleeding
Level of consciousness changes
Multiple IV solutions, lines, and rates
Site complications
Continuous bladder irrigation
Transferring patients
Family visits
Codes
Reports to floor nurses.[34]

The use of simulation standardizes the stimuli to which students are exposed.

SUMMARY

The National League for Nursing has identified core competencies for nurse educators that include the implementation of advanced technologies to support the teaching–learning process. The League has also unveiled a Web site to facilitate the integration of simulation technology into nursing education curricula. Its aim is to encourage nurse educators to develop expertise in simulation education modalities. This Web site has nine online courses with interactive exercises and video clips of simulation scenarios and interactive programs. In addition, there are public forums to share information, an annotated bibliography of simulation articles, and a resource center with information on funding opportunities, vendors, and simulation centers.[35,36] Although more research is needed on high-fidelity simulation in nursing, simulation can be an exciting application of advanced technology in nursing education. It is rapidly becoming state-of-the-art in teaching nursing because it can bridge the gap between classroom instruction and the unpredictable clinical area.

REFERENCES

1. Daley K. Making simulation real: the integration journey. In: Programs and abstracts of the Laerdal Simulation Users Group Conference. Ledyard (CT); 2006.
2. Gaberson KB, Oermann MH. Clinical teaching strategies in nursing. 2nd edition. New York: Springer Pub; 2007.
3. Morton PG. Academic education. Creating a laboratory that simulates the critical care environment. Crit Care Nurse 1996;16(6):76–81.
4. Jeffries PR. National league for nursing. Simulation in nursing education: from conceptualization to evaluation. New York: National League for Nursing; 2007. p. 168. Available at: http://www.laerdal.com/document.asp?subnodeid527721661. Accessed May 7, 2008.
5. Parr MB, Sweeney NM. Use of human patient simulation in an undergraduate critical care course. Crit Care Nurs Q 2006;29(3):188–98.
6. Starkweather AR, Kardong-Edgren S. Diffusion of innovation: embedding simulation into nursing curricula. Int J Nurs Educ Scholarsh 2008;5(1):Article 13.
7. Ackermann A. Education for nursing students using human patient simulation. In: Programs and abstracts of the Nursing Education on the Move: Technology, Creativity and Innovation. Philadelphia; 2006.
8. Oren T. Future of modeling and simulation: some development areas. Available at: http://64.233.169.104/search?q=cache:eAdyEwzRqsEJ:www.site.uottawa.ca/~oren/pubs/D85-Shanghai-Ethical.pdf+negative+consequences+of+simulation&;hl=en&ct=clnk&cd=2&gl=us. Accessed May 14, 2008.
9. Jones AP, Homer JB, Murphy DL, et al. Understanding diabetes population dynamics through simulation modeling and experimentation. Am J Public Health 2006;96(3):488–94.
10. History of flight simulation. Available at: http://www.acecombatsix.com/flight_Simulations/index.html. Accessed May 14, 2008.
11. A brief history of aircraft flight simulation (flight training). Available at: http://homepage.ntlworld.com/bleep/SimHist3.html. Accessed May 14, 2008.
12. Lupien AE. Innovative teaching strategies in nursing and related health professions. 4th edition. Sudbury (MA): Jones and Bartlett Publishers; 2007.
13. Hovancsek MT. Using simulation in nursing education. In: Jeffries PR, editor. Simulation in nursing education. New York: National League for Nursing; 2007. p. 1–9.
14. Medical Education Technologies. Medical Education Technologies Inc Web site. Available at: http://www.meti.com/products_ps_istan.htm2008.

15. Chambers K. Simulation in nursing education: the basics. In: Programs and abstracts of the Laerdal Simulation Users Group Conference. Ledyard (CT): 2006.
16. Mitchell J. New grad RNs in the virtual care unit—taking critical care education to new heights. In: Programs and abstracts of the Nursing Education on the Move: Technology, Creativity and Innovation. Philadelphia; 2006.
17. Henneman EA, Cunningham H, Roche JP, et al. Human patient simulation: teaching students to provide safe care. Nurse Educ 2007;32(5):212–7.
18. Lamond D, Crow R, Chase J, et al. Information sources used in decision making: considerations for simulation development. Int J Nurs Stud 1996;33(1):47–57.
19. Preventing medication errors: quality chasm series—Institute of Medicine. Available at: http://www.iom.edu/CMS/3809/22526/35939.aspx. Accessed July 10, 2008.
20. Henneman EA, Cunningham H. Using clinical simulation to teach patient safety in an acute/critical care nursing course. Nurse Educ 2005;30(4):172–7.
21. Lerman LG. The simulated patient. Public Health Rep 1996;111(2):133–4.
22. Weis PA, Guyton-Simmons J. A computer simulation for teaching critical thinking skills. Nurse Educ 1998;23(2):30–3.
23. Ravert P. An integrative review of computer-based simulation in the education process. Comput Inform Nurs 2002;20(5):203–8.
24. Woody G, Cherry. Simulation: intravenous catheter insertion. Submitted for review.
25. Roberson DW, Neil JA, Bryant E. A malodorous wound simulation study. Ostomy/Wound Management 2008;54(8):36–43.
26. Young JS, Dubose JE, Hedrick TL, et al. The use of "war games" to evaluate performance of students and residents in basic clinical scenarios: a disturbing analysis. J Trauma 2007;63(3):556–64.
27. Pothier PK. Create a low-cost tracheotomy model for suctioning simulation. Nurse Educ 2006;31(5):192–4.
28. Persaud D. Mentoring the new graduate perioperative nurse: valuable retention strategy. AORN J 2008;87(6):1173–9.
29. Spencer KW. Patient simulation to enhance patient safety. Plast Surg Nurs 2006; 26(4):195–7.
30. Anderson M, LeFlore J. Playing it safe: simulated team training in the OR. AORN J 2008;87(4):772–9.
31. WISER-WISER home. Available at: http://www.wiser.pitt.edu/. Accessed July 10, 2008.
32. Simulation in nursing education—UT Arlington. Available at: http://www.uta.edu/nursing/simulation/smart_hospital.php. Accessed May 7, 2008.
33. Nyswaner A. "Driver's ed" for the OR nurse. RN 2007;70(3):45–8.
34. O'Connor AB, National league for nursing. Clinical instruction and evaluation: a teaching resource. Boston: Jones and Bartlett Publishers; 2001.
35. National league for nursing. Available at: http://sirc.nln.org. Accessed June, 17 2008, 2008.
36. King CJ, Moseley S, Hindenlang B, et al. Limited use of the human patient simulator by nurse faculty: An intervention program designed to increase use. Int J Nurs Educ Scholarsh 2008;5(1):1–17.

Creating a Place for Perioperative Nursing in Graduate Programs

Nancy Girard, PhD, RN, FAAN

KEYWORDS

- Graduate education • Certification • Advanced practice
- Preceptors • Faculty

Perioperative nurses, as with those who work in any area of nursing, need advanced education if they are to advance in their careers. The term *graduate* is sometimes used to describe students who graduate from nursing school. In this article, "graduate student" means one enrolled in higher education in a formal academic setting, such as a university. In most hospitals and health care institutions today, nurses holding diploma certificates, associate degrees, and baccalaureate degrees provide most of the bedside or direct nursing care. These nurses are the front line of care and are invaluable. In the operating room, they most frequently serve as registered nurse (RN) circulators or they run a product line, such as orthopedics or neurosurgery. Many institutions, however, now require the Bachelor of Science in Nursing (BSN) degree for lower management positions, depending on the size and state in which the institution is located; further, such institutions now require the Master of Science in Nursing (MSN) or a similar graduate degree for higher level or unit leadership. More and more, hospitals now also require the MSN or an equivalent degree for management positions.

Further, hospitals and health care institutions now often require an area of specialization for advanced practice. These nurses are generically called advanced practice registered nurses (APRNs). Specific APRN roles include clinical nurse specialist (CNS), nurse practitioner (NP), and certified registered nurse anesthetist (CRNA). An even newer role that now requires an MSN or equivalent master's degree is that of the clinical nurse leader (CNL). The CNL is a generalist but is not considered to be an advanced practice nurse.

GRADUATE PROGRAMS

Graduate nursing programs usually impose the prerequisite of an undergraduate degree for entrance. There are some exceptions for RNs who lack the baccalaureate degree in nursing. For example, some universities offer a "fast track" program in which

Department of Acute Nursing Care, University of Texas Health Science Center at San Antonio, San Antonio, TX 78229, USA
E-mail address: ngirard2@satx.rr.com

Perioperative Nursing Clinics 4 (2009) 113–120
doi:10.1016/j.cpen.2009.01.004
1556-7931/09/$ – see front matter © 2009 Elsevier Inc. All rights reserved.

a student with a degree other than in nursing can matriculate to secure an MSN degree. Still other institutions offer the option of RN-to-MSN or even RN-to–Doctor of Philosophy (PhD) programs. In these programs, the core undergraduate nursing degree is built into the program and the BSN or MSN degree is given on graduation. Other options may be available at select schools.

All schools that offer credible graduate degrees must be accredited by recognized bodies, normally as a requisite of state law. The main organizations that accredit graduate nursing programs are the Commission on Collegiate Nursing Education (CCNE) and the National League for Nursing Accrediting Commission (NLNAC). The CCNE is the accepted accrediting body that normally accredits graduate nursing programs, whereas the NLNAC is the recognized entity that usually accredits undergraduate, associate, and diploma programs. Between the two, more than 330 master's degree programs have achieved accreditation.[1] There are other approval groups under which nursing schools must work, including regional, professional, and state agencies for higher education. Some are highly prescriptive as to the nursing curriculum needed for each program, and these bodies must approve any new offerings. For example, to offer an approved new major, such as perioperative nursing, in a graduate program at universities in Texas, a detailed proposal and full curriculum must be approved by no less than three, and possibly four, separate bodies: (1) the school's graduate curriculum committee; (2) if associated with a health science center, the graduate school; (3) the state's Board of Nursing; and (4) the Texas Higher Education Coordinating Board.

This complex process of programmatic approval can take up to a year and a half to secure full approval, plus perhaps another full year to advertise and to enroll enough students to begin the program. A private school may not have as many of the processes to negotiate as does a public one and can offer more flexibility, but a private program must still obtain full accreditation by a recognized body and other entities as well.

The new program's proposed curriculum must contain specific content, a required number of credit hours, and a specific time within which full-time students must complete all requirements. Graduating students must also pass national certification examinations at the end of their schooling. Depending on the state in which the desired program is located, entrance requirements necessarily vary somewhat. Past academic grades are usually a determining factor for acceptance to a program, with an average of B or higher. Generally, graduate program entrance requirements include all previous schools' course transcripts in addition to scores from the Management Aptitude Test, the Graduate Record Examination, or both. Minimum required scores on these examinations vary from school to school and from year to year. Other than all national, state, and school requirements, each school may have additional or waiver requirements so that the interested student needs to research requirements for his or her school(s) of choice. For example, if one were to apply to enroll in an acute care nurse practitioner (ACNP) program, the applicant might need to have a minimum of 2 years' experience working in a critical care environment (note that work in the operating room ordinarily does not count toward meeting such an experience requirement).

MAJORS THAT CAN INCORPORATE PERIOPERATIVE NURSING CONTENT

The most common majors that perioperative nurses seek are advanced practice, administration, and CRNA. A new major now offered more throughout the country is the CNL. The CNL, as mentioned previously, is a generalist but is not considered to be an advanced practice nurse.[2] An APRN must hold a master's degree or higher, must have completed an approved program, and must hold national certification.

Today, NPs must practice within their scope of practice. For example, in the past, hospitals hired family NPs for acute care areas. Now, however, these nurses must be ACNPs if they work in the operating room, intensive care, medical-surgical, or emergency areas. Advanced practice also includes the CNS in critical care or medical-surgical nursing.

Perioperative CNS programs are rare today, although a few existed in the past. The military still offers this curriculum.[3] Some schools that had this major in the past no longer offer it for several reasons: low numbers of students, lack of support of the school, minimal local employment opportunities, and no advanced certification examinations specifically for perioperative nurses. Without such formal recognition accorded by national advanced certification testing, schools cannot produce students who could secure certification, and would thus be impossibly limited in their employment opportunities.

In addition to APRN education, other programs in which perioperative nurses are often interested include nursing administration or management programs that pair well with perioperative needs. Some schools offer a combined MSN/Master of Business Administration degree. Educational majors are becoming more prevalent today. The need for new faculty is critical, and the educational major may be the most important graduate major today. General curriculum and instructional theories and concepts often can be used in any educational situation, from the formal academic arena to staff development education. CNL programs are growing in number. CNL students are prepared to serve in leadership, informatics, practice, and other roles needed by health care institutions today, notwithstanding that they are neither certified nor prepared to serve in CNS or other APRN positions.

MINORS THAT CAN INCORPORATE PERIOPERATIVE NURSING CONTENT

Most schools require 6 hours of a minor in addition to electives. Minors differ from school to school, but minors are usually two 3-hour courses that provide 6 credit hours. A minor can be anything that the school thinks is important to the community and to students. Minor proposals must meet curriculum committee approval and are offered sequentially every semester. The student then graduates with a major and a minor, which show up on grade transcripts. This may prove helpful in obtaining specific career positions.

Minors can be a condensed form of any major, such as management or education. They can also center on subject area, such as geriatric or informatics. A perioperative focus can be enhanced in any minor, just as in any major. The student must demonstrate to the professor that he or she can complete all course requirements using a perioperative focus and negotiate for consideration at the beginning of each semester.

ELECTIVES

Schools also usually require students to complete a set number of elective credit hours. The most common requirement is 6 to 9 credit hours and is intended to satisfy student interests or to increase depth in a specific career trajectory, such as orthopedic or renal nursing. Basic perioperative electives are usually one 3-hour course given in the undergraduate program; they are seldom offered as a minor in graduate programs.

Depending on the school, students can take an elective course as independent study (IS). With an IS elective, a perioperative graduate student would first identify a supportive faculty member, presumably an educator particularly knowledgeable in perioperative nursing, and then would obtain permission to work with that faculty member for credit hours ranging from 1 to 4 credit hours per course. IS electives can be tailored specifically for the perioperative student and might include anything not already given in a formal course.

The IS course goal might be to deepen the student's knowledge or understanding in clinical practice, research, administration, or education. If such opportunities exist in a particular graduate program, the student first would have to develop written course objectives, also addressing content that the student proposes to learn; outline how the faculty member would evaluate student knowledge; and, finally, define where clinical experiences, if any, would occur. The faculty member would then have to preapprove the course description, submit it for approval to the appropriate school committee, and, if it is approved, oversee student instruction throughout the semester.

Examples of possible IS courses are numerous. They run from learning data entry for research to studying clinical procedures for patient outcomes and from translating learned concepts into practical clinical practice to broadening and deepening knowledge in specific areas, such as anatomy or neurosurgery. A simple Web search can provide the interested student with a broad range of additional information about schools of particular interest.[4]

BARRIERS TO INCREASING PERIOPERATIVE NURSING CONTENT

Barriers exist to increasing perioperative nursing content in graduate programs on two sides, the academic and clinical sides, when one considers how to implement content in any graduate programs. First, there are commonsensical problems that both sides face, such as, simply, time. Faculty and clinicians are already burdened by heavy outside time commitments, not to mention often intense and routinely full work days. Both may feel compelled to minimize or simply to deny what little added time they still have to give to others outside the existing environment. That reluctance to further time commitments includes those to new graduate IS students intent on developing perioperative skills.

There may also be a general lack of perceived awareness of need by many faculty and clinicians for such additions, not to mention real institutional financial constraints that seem to preclude or substantially limit any expansion of existing programs or educational opportunities. In addition, experience suggests that a group prefers to remain in its comfort zone, or, some might say, tunnel, and does not expand beyond it if given a choice. More collaboration in some communities between academia and health care providers tends to disprove these barriers, and the outcomes produced by working together are immensely beneficial and profitable in many ways to both.[5]

As for barriers more specific to academia, some major factors that tend to prevent the introduction of more perioperative nursing content into graduate programs are a severe lack of qualified, not to mention interested, faculty. Faculty members who support perioperative nursing must be ready to advocate the specialty to their colleagues and to promote the perioperative environment for clinical experiences. The biggest academic barrier, one hard to admit, remains an overarching ignorance: most faculties remain woefully unaware of the importance of perioperative nursing.

Indeed, some faculty members do not recognize the perioperative specialty to be nursing at all, and those who profess such negative views can affect other faculty members. Such "nay sayers" may also tend to steer students toward other specialties, more often than not their own. Students in graduate schools who come as perioperative nurses may thus be moved into other areas considered more valuable, and by the time they graduate, perioperative nursing may no longer be their prime objective.

As for clinicians, there may be a sheer lack of understanding of the academic process and the boundaries within which it must operate. Clinicians historically underestimate the workload and value of a faculty member and consider the old saying to be true that "those who can do, those who can't teach." Nothing could be further from the truth in both instances. Unless the collaborating school in question is a private school that can alter curriculum easily and quickly, trying to mandate the inclusion of perioperative nursing by the faculty fails more often than not.

There is also a prevailing lack of available preceptors in clinical areas. Many, if not most, staff nurses educationally hold the BSN degree or less. Accreditation requirements for most schools include clinical requirements specifying that a student must be precepted by a clinician with an academic degree or degrees higher than that of the student, in addition to having expertise in the area of practice. Even if faculty members try to circumvent this requirement by serving, on paper, as the major preceptor and using outstanding clinicians in the hospital, whatever their educational level, the fact remains that truly qualified preceptors remain scarce and in great demand by faculty. Worse, there is ongoing competition between CNS, administration, and NP faculty for the same person at the same clinical site. A manager or APRN in the perioperative area has skills and knowledge that can be used in many arenas and can serve as a preceptor for most of the majors offered. These preceptors are thus overused and quickly become burned out, further increasing the lack of qualified preceptors.

As stated previously, no certification or advanced practice examination exists for perioperative nurses, and this omission raises its own "catch 22" puzzle. Those who run the perioperative certification examination (Certified Nurse in the Operating Room) assert that there is not enough demand to construct an advanced practice examination. Students who are interested cannot major in perioperative nursing because there is no advanced certification test, and thus must opt for another major. It was not always so.

For many years, the University of Texas Health Science Center at San Antonio (UTHSCSA) offered the perioperative CNS major in its graduate program. These nurse graduates went on to serve admirably as outstanding managers and APRNs in public and military environments. On graduation, however, there remained the serious problem that those graduate students needed to take a certification examination for the APRN designator. The only examination that fit the need was the medical-surgical CNS examination. The certification board soon decreed that these graduate students did not have the requisite medical-surgical curricular content needed (although their curricular content had been entirely surgical). The result was that the school had to fight with the certification board over student eligibility annually. Finally, the school determined that without an advanced certification examination in the specialty, it could no longer offer the perioperative major and discontinued that offering.

WHAT PERIOPERATIVE NURSES CAN DO

Notwithstanding, clinical nurses today can do many things to facilitate the incorporation of significant perioperative content into a nursing program. They can help to forge strong relationships by collaborating with nursing faculty on projects, they can serve as preceptors, and they can work actively with motivated graduate students. It is invaluable for a graduate student to see and work with excellent role models in clinical practice whether the clinician acts as a clinical educator, APRN, or administrator. If a graduate student can participate in a project that the hospital or institution wants and needs, that helps both organizations: the graduate school and the institution. This participation may include attendance at committee meetings, review of data, and even the study of financial records. If the participating student needs these activities to complete a project, the student can readily sign a confidentiality agreement with the preceptor and institution, as needed, so that the hospital is comfortable in sharing all necessary information for a realistic and valuable learning experience.

APRNs, in addition to nurse administrators or managers, can volunteer to share their professional experiences with graduate nursing students. They can also agree to present case studies, to serve on panels for discussion, and even to present a guest lecture. Doing so can enhance student knowledge and awareness of experiences that they are likely to encounter once they begin to work in their new role after graduation. Many schools appoint qualified clinical nurses who want to contribute to the school and assist with student education to nonfunded positions as adjunct faculty.

To increase a fuller understanding of perioperative nursing, clinical nurses can present information at a partner school of nursing. An opportune time for doing so might be during Perioperative Nurses' Week. Some constructive examples of such sharing come to mind. Clinical nurses might prepare provocative posters about quality improvement projects that ultimately aim to stimulate project ideas for graduate students and their course assignments. Clinical nurses might also present informatively about perioperative nurses' community involvement, such as giving tours of the operating room for children and families.

Some examples of how hospitals generally can help themselves and the education of nurses for their facilities are to offer work-study programs or to provide grants to schools to develop and offer courses just for the hospital. Such a course might be a bridge course for undergraduates. Bridge courses provide the opportunity for students in their last semester to work on a unit of their choice, such as the operating room, while still students. The charge nurse and the faculty member need to interview interested students, because enrollment in the bridge course depends on a successful 3-month placement. Benefits for the student are elective credit, actual work experience, and an opportunity to see if this is indeed what he or she wants for a career.

For the hospital, bridge courses allow nurses to see if the potential new hire would fit within their unit and contribute to the environment and patient care. If all turns out well, the hospital may hire the student at graduation and orientation time greatly decreases. The new graduate is ready to hit the floor running.

Although bridge courses are mostly for undergraduates, there is the opportunity for graduate students to work within the course as a beginning educator or APRN. Another valuable result is the potential to hire faculty for part-time clinical work. This allows the faculty member to obtain needed clinical hours for recertification and to maintain skills. It benefits the hospital further because it may secure a skilled consultant, researcher, or educator inexpensively at a fraction of the cost of a full-time employee.

WHAT FACULTY MEMBERS CAN DO

A school of nursing can do many things to promote perioperative nursing specifically and nursing in general. First, however, it must meet a key requirement: to identify that faculty member (or members) who is a perioperative nurse and who is willing to work within the boundaries of the university and the school to incorporate needed apt curricular content into existing courses. This is critical, because extant courses are most often crammed with required content. Adding more hours to the curriculum for any specialty is therefore not easily done.

Hiring clinically competent and qualified APRN educators is an ongoing concern for schools, given that active practitioners normally enjoy higher salaries than do educators. Joint or part-time appointments, especially for APRNs, greatly facilitate more effective work forces in academia. These faculties also must work directly with patients to be recertified. Often, these faculty members find themselves in a difficult situation. MSN-prepared faculty can teach undergraduate students and usually have a heavy clinical teaching load. They also may teach students who major in an APRN program. Thus, if they practice, it must be on their day off. If they do not practice, they lose their certification and are not eligible to teach or to practice. If a hospital were to offer a practitioner a 20% to 50% part-time clinical position, it would bring teaching and practice expertise, both enormously valuable, to the clinical institution.

Nurses with a PhD end degree teach in graduate programs and do academic research. They can bring their research knowledge and expertise to the hospital, can opt to work with staff to learn quality improvement strategies and clinical research, can help with the translation of research, and can offer innovative writing and other workshops as needed by the hospital. Such educator-clinicians can also work with midlevel managers to provide a healthy workplace, to develop better leadership strategies, to address working with difficult staff, and to explore other topics like finance and informatics. Just as clinicians might create engaging posters for the school, expert faculty can present their research and projects to the hospital during Nurses' or Perioperative Nurses' Week.

Likewise, schools can offer electives useful to graduate students and add perioperative content to established courses. Examples of work problems and their solutions and case studies that incorporate perioperative content may be easily inserted into lectures and discussions. Many courses can include aspects of perioperative nursing. For example, in the administration major, perioperative students can be assigned to work with an operating room director or surgical services vice-president to gain experience in the area of focus. Every assignment in the course then focuses on the perioperative setting, staff, problems, and solutions. School papers, projects, and dissertations may then have perioperative nursing as a focus. Educators can also agree to monitor IS that focuses on surgical topics and to identify perioperative care preceptors through the local Association of PeriOperative Registered Nurses (AORN) chapter.

Other suggestions for faculty include forging strong partnerships, establishing core professional and clinical competencies, and collaborating with other health care professionals. For example, the UTHSCSA Acute Nursing Care (ANC) Department teamed with the University Medical School and School of Allied Health to offer a collaborative advanced anatomy course. The course was mandatory for medical students and physician assistants, and it was offered as an elective to CNS and ACNP students. There was an associated cadaver laboratory if the nursing student wished to participate.

The ANC Department also created a relationship with the Department of Anesthesiology. This school was expert in using simulation in teaching and had acquired expensive manikins and technology. The ANC Department Chair wrote and secured a grant that enabled the Department of Anesthesiology to include graduate ACNP student nurses in simulated learning of advanced resuscitation, intubation, wound closure, chest tube placement, and many other related skills. An incidental but important and ongoing benefit of these collaborative partnership activities was heightened team building and a deeper understanding of the participants' respective skills and professional goals.

SUMMARY

Adding perioperative nursing content to graduate school courses requires the active cooperation and interest of our academic and clinical institutions. Our schools prepare students for increasingly vital roles in our communities, just as our health care institutions provide life-preserving and life-enhancing services to the nation. Once we recognize the need for expert perioperative nurses with MSN degrees, our schools must necessarily give serious consideration to helping our nation and communities by educating for those roles. Although many ideas are offered in this article, there are probably as many or more solutions being tried that we have yet to recognize. Those involved in innovative educational methods and creative teaching and practice must be willing to share their ideas, plans, and solutions. It is hoped, in that light, that some of the ideas given here stimulate further thought and serious action to increase the number of perioperative nurses with advanced degrees. The surgical world has become so complicated that promoting perioperative graduate education is ultimately likely to prove invaluable to our nation and the world.

REFERENCES

1. Dracup K. Master's nursing programs. Available at: http://www.aacn.nche.edu/education/nurse_ed/MSNArticle.htm. Accessed November 19, 2008.
2. White paper AORN. Clinical nurse leader. Available at: http://www.aorn.org/docs_assets/55B250E0-9779-5C0D-1DDC8177C9B4C8EB/F2DD79C6-A207-7FF3-631E7597738D778F/Ref_Clinical_Nurse_Leader_-_REVISED__2_.pdf. 2006. Accessed November 19, 2008.
3. USU Graduate School of Nursing. Available at: http://www.usuhs.mil/gsn/cns/cnsprogram.html. Accessed November 19, 2008.
4. Masters in nursing. Available at: http://www.mastersinnursing.com. Accessed November 19, 2008.
5. Girard NJ. Perioperative education—perspective from the think tank. AORN J 2004;80:827–35, 838.

Improving Diversity in Nursing Education

Lana M. deRuyter, PhD, RN*, Melanie O. Leroy, PhD, RN, CRNP

KEYWORDS

- Minority • Diversity • Culture care • Nursing education
- Associate degree • Baccalaureate degree

Significant and ongoing discussions continue on how to improve diversity in the health care workforce. The number of minorities entering the workforce in health care-related fields remains lower than in the general population.[1] As proposed by The Sullivan Commission, increasing the number of minority graduate nurses may help to lessen the shortage of nurses in underserved areas and to improve health care delivery to underserved populations, who notes "We know that minority physicians, dentists, and nurses are more likely to serve minority and medically underserved populations, yet there continues to be a severe shortage of minorities in the health professions."[2]

The initiative to increase minority graduate nurses is a reflection of what has been understood for decades. Demographics in the United States continue to change, with substantial increases across multiple ethnic minorities. It is anticipated that these minority populations are likely to continue to grow rapidly. What is apparent and problematic is that diversity within the health care work force is failing to keep pace with this burgeoning growth of America's ethnic minorities.

At present, African-American nursing students who enter colleges and universities are at risk for attrition and failure to complete their nursing degrees.[3,4] The challenge looming for educators is to identify barriers to the success of African-American nursing students, along with strategies to improve their retention and academic success in nursing schools. Some known barriers to success include discrimination, feelings of isolation, loneliness, and the perceived experience of being "other" (ie, feeling different). Kosowski and colleagues[4] highlighted the impact of being a minority student in a majoritarian culture, that is, one in which white students and faculty are in a majority numerically. Other barriers focus on the challenges minority students face with testing, comparatively poor secondary preparation for higher education, and financial constraints. In addition, American nursing educational institutions lack substantial minority faculties able to serve as role models and leaders for minority nursing students.

Nursing Department, Delaware County Community College, 901 S. Media Line Road, Media, PA 19063, USA.
* Corresponding author.
E-mail address: lderuyte@dccc.edu (L.M. deRuyter).

Perioperative Nursing Clinics 4 (2009) 121–129
doi:10.1016/j.cpen.2009.01.005
1556-7931/09/$ – see front matter © 2009 Elsevier Inc. All rights reserved.

Examples of successful interventions include hiring faculty whose designated role is to work with minority students and to help them feel "part of the group." This faculty member assists struggling students academically. Also needed is the provision of additional support services to help struggling African-American students succeed academically.[5,6] Such support services include helping minority students with time management issues, study skills, and note-taking and test-taking skills.

Two nurse researchers were interested in identifying issues and strategies that could improve the success rate for African-American nursing students. One study focused on baccalaureate students and registered nurses, whereas the second study focused on associate degree nursing students, identifying their culture, care, education, and experiences. This article discusses the results of these two studies.

ISSUES AND STRATEGIES: AFRICAN-AMERICAN BACCALAUREATE NURSING STUDENTS

Taken from the perspectives of registered nurses and baccalaureate students, the first study identified strategies that have the potential to improve retention and academic success for African-American nursing students. Nine baccalaureate students and three registered nurses participated in a qualitative descriptive study designed to answer the research question reflected previously in this article. Six themes emerged from data analysis of the participants' perceptions of factors that may be faculty or student driven and that can influence academic success. These themes are: (1) being accessible to students who need academic help, (2) conveying a willingness to assist students, (3) encouraging students in ways that help to build self-confidence, (4) struggling as an African-American student from perceived unequal treatment, (5) needing to experience a sense of belonging to succeed, and (6) struggling to achieve academic success.

In the qualitative review, themes 4 through 6 ascended in importance in that they developed the context in which the first three themes should be viewed. These three themes derived from examples of the struggles African-American students endure while working toward a nursing degree. Theme 4, struggling as an African-American student from perceived unequal treatment, emerged from personal examples of students focused on inequality in grading, variations in acceptable clinical and classroom behavior, and inflexibility by faculty.

Educational racism is addressed in the literature, and the nursing profession has long been viewed as one for white women.[7–9] The existence of racial prejudice within nursing curricula has also been identified by other nursing scholars.[8,10,11] Majority faculty may not accord value to the perception of unequal treatment, leading to a lack of academic success, and many majority faculty deny the existence of personal bias or prejudice. Yet, the fact remains that these study participants perceived that there was unequal treatment on the part of majority faculty. Tucker-Allen and Long[6] identified the impact of faculty attitudes on academic success of minority nursing students. Identifying personal bias and being sensitive to the perception of unequal treatment were noted as helpful to nurse educators who wished to improve academic outcomes and graduation rates for minority nursing students. Conversely, denying that those perceptions exist tended to perpetuate experiences discussed by the participants in this study.

The participants in this study also expressed a sense of isolation and loneliness associated with being different from majority students in their nursing classes. At the same time, theme 5, needing to experience a sense of belonging to succeed, developed from the acknowledgment that having, for example, a peer group with whom to study helped student participants to achieve academic success.

Study participants suggested that they felt alienated and that it was easy to feel insecure because of the small numbers of African-American nursing students in their classes. Sensing differences from many others in the group can lead to feelings of isolation and alienation on the part of the minority student. This sense of "otherness" has the potential to be a barrier to success for minority nursing students.[12] The need for a sense of belonging to succeed reflects published data that suggest minority nursing students feel a sense of aloneness and isolation and that these feelings impede academic success.[3,5,6]

The participants in this study also identified the importance of study groups for academic success. Certainly, study partners helped with understanding challenging academic materials; the participants, however, tended more to note that members of their study groups became close and were viewed as family. The support the participants received was more than help with understanding theoretic content. Study group members supported and encouraged each other, giving members a sense of fellowship and belonging that counteracted the perception of somehow being other. Ultimately, the data suggested that the sense of fellowship and belonging that occurs as a result of being part of a group bound by mutual goals was a motivating factor that led to academic success.

The final theme, struggling to achieve academic success, identified the workload associated with the nursing curriculum and how transitioning into the junior year of college was the most challenging for participants. Many participants discussed how the rigor of the nursing program came as a surprise. The theoretic and clinical work created an academic burden that the participants in this study felt unprepared to meet. The intensity of nursing programs with respect to workload has previously been identified in the literature as a barrier to success.[9,10]

In addition, testing methodology in nursing programs often incorporates "higher level thinking" questions that are objective in nature. Many study participants reported that they had not encountered these "higher level" multiple choice questions before nursing school. The issue with higher level multiple choice testing is related to the challenge that minority students have with respect to the comparative inability to excel in standardized testing.[13] In addition, participants in this study worried about what would be on tests and discussed how test questions did not seem to reflect theoretic content covered in class. These concerns led to high levels of anxiety at the time of testing, further impairing the ability to perform successfully.

This study identified three forms of faculty intervention that, in the opinion of the participants, had the potential to improve academic outcomes for minority nursing students. They were (1) more open faculty access, (2) greater faculty help, and (3) increased faculty encouragement. It is recognized that although these three themes seem to be distinct, there is necessarily some overlap (ie, all three enhance the student-faculty relationship). In addition, although one may argue legitimately that these issues are not unique to African-American nursing students, one must nevertheless view the data from the perspective of the ethnic minority student, who, in this study, reported feeling different and apart and reported the perceived experience of unequal treatment based on race.

The first form of faculty intervention, focused on more open access to faculty, has two unique extensions. First is the issue of time and availability on the part of the student and how difficult it is for many to carve out time to meet with faculty during regularly scheduled but often limited office hours. The second extension to the first form of faculty intervention reflects the willingness of faculty to adjust their posted hours and personal schedules to meet with time-pressed minority students. Many study participants were forced to juggle classes, work, and pressing family issues and found it challenging, if not impossible, to find time to meet with faculty.

Study participants' perceptions of faculty attitudes as they asked for special consideration was important with respect to their degree of self-confidence as they approached faculty for additional instruction during non–office-hour times. Lack of faculty access may be viewed as a barrier to success. Nursing is a caring profession, and, as such, nursing faculty need to demonstrate a caring attitude when attempting to meet the needs of African-American nursing students. Being accessible and available for all students is essential if one is to develop positive student-faculty relationships that have the potential to motivate and to guide students toward retention and academic success.

Another issue identified by study participants was the willingness of faculty to assist students. Overwhelmingly, participants recognized their need for faculty intervention when they were struggling with grades and content and knew they should go to faculty for assistance. By conveying a willingness to help students, faculty members were seen as providing a foundation on which to establish a positive student-faculty relationship. Participants viewed faculty who readily met with students as worthy and memorable. Nursing faculty members are in a unique position to help students achieve academic success by providing added and requisite support to struggling students. Some areas in which faculty were seen as particularly helpful were (1) pointing out time management strategies, (2) helping students to organize papers, and (3) making suggestions to improve study habits. In addition, many students came to faculty hoping to gain a greater understanding of difficult and challenging concepts.

The nursing literature supports the need for additional support services for minority nursing students.[5] Positive faculty attitudes and assistance, coupled with support services, can guide students toward academic success.[6,10,14,15]

The final theme from this study focused on the need students seem to have to hear words of encouragement from their professors. Participants discussed the need to be reassured that they had the ability to be successful, and they were encouraged when faculty told them that they could succeed. Faculty reassurance tended to build self-esteem, which, in turn, led to a sense of empowerment and success. This allowed students to overcome psychologic barriers to success, thus providing internal tools with which to build themselves up and to move forward toward their goals.[6,12]

Participants in the study made recurring and compelling comments that failed to reach methodologic saturation. Students repeatedly noted their own personal determination, but, likewise, raised the issue of the negative impact that the lack of African-American nursing faculty to serve as mentors and role models has on them. Notwithstanding this lack, personal determination motivated some study participants to find help and assistance to succeed and to achieve their academic goals.

Minority students felt challenged by the lack of diversity among nursing faculty. African-American faculty understand what it is like to be an ethnic minority in the United States and are able to relate to the unequal treatment experienced by African Americans in this society. This problem is an issue that cannot be resolved until more African-American nurses graduate from nursing programs and pursue advanced degrees.

Nursing is a dynamic profession that has changed dramatically based on societal demands. Nursing programs strive to educate independent thinkers, patient advocates, and patient educators. As such, nursing programs bear a responsibility to maintain the highest level of commitment to the profession and to society as a whole. In one respect, the nursing profession has failed to keep up with the changes occurring in society. Nursing simply has failed to graduate African-American registered nurses in substantial numbers, and workforce diversity continues to be hugely problematic despite decades of acknowledging this growing issue. The participants in this study spoke at length about their perceptions of unequal treatment from nursing faculty, and it is now necessary for nursing faculty to recognize those perceptions and attempt to understand the impact they have on academic success.

Faculty must also look within and be open to seeing internal bias or prejudice that may influence their interactions with ethnic minority students. Faculty open to such self-examination may choose to attend faculty development sessions geared toward diversity and the privilege of being white in a majoritarian society. The expressions of these participants are validated in the literature, and faculty are encouraged to read the data supporting the perceptions of unequal treatment among African-American nursing students.

The primary themes of the study, in which participants asked for faculty availability, willingness to help, and encouragement, reflect students' desire to become integral to the student-teacher relationship. Students must recognize their responsibility in forming that relationship and be prepared to keep appointments and follow through with suggestions provided to guide them toward academic success. The obligations of teacher and student should be presented at the time of orientation to the nursing program. Reality sometimes requires students to reschedule or forego some preset activity so that they have the chance to meet with faculty. Students were encouraged when they heard faculty tell them that they could succeed. Encouragement leads to self-confidence, and self-confidence leads to success. Students who feel insecure or lack confidence may gain an advantage by hearing that they can be successful.

ISSUES AND STRATEGIES: AFRICAN-AMERICAN ASSOCIATE DEGREE NURSING STUDENTS

The second study was a qualitative ethnonursing study designed to discover the cultural care education and experiences of African-American students in predominantly Euro-American associate degree nursing programs. Leininger's Culture Care Diversity and Universality Theory was the conceptual framework for this study. Interviews with 28 nursing students from eight associate degree nursing programs located in southeastern Pennsylvania and southern New Jersey were the source of the data. From this study, 14 major categories, eight patterns, and three common themes emerged. The common themes were (1) care, understanding, and spirituality by family, friends, and faculty are essential for meaningful educational experiences for African-American students; (2) for African-American students, professional and generic health and illness beliefs are holistic concepts incorporated into all aspects of life, including a professional nursing education; and (3) care expressed through social interactions, financial support, resources, and scheduling is viewed as significant to beneficial educational outcomes for African-American students.

The second study developed a conceptual model (**Fig. 1**) to illustrate the relation between these three common thematic concepts. Together, all three themes provide a beginning insight into the daily lives, expectations, experiences, values, and beliefs of African-American students in associate degree programs that are predominantly Euro-American (ie, white).

The study postulated that discovery of the cultural life ways, beliefs, and educational experiences of African-American students in predominantly Euro-American associate degree programs would provide data that associate degree nursing programs and nurse educators could use to develop more culturally sensitive and congruent educational care. If nursing curricula were taught in a culturally sensitive and congruent manner, this, arguably, would promote more meaningful educational experiences

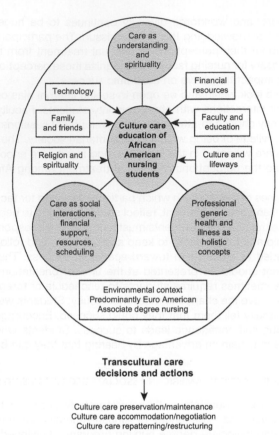

Fig. 1. deRuyter's model of culture care education. (*From* deRuyter LM. Culture care education and experiences of African American students in predominantly Euro American associate degree nursing programs [dissertation]. UMI Microform 3303013. Ann Arbor, MI: ProQuest Information and Learning Company, 2008; with permission.)

and ultimately help to improve retention and graduation rates of African-American students.

A primary concept that clearly emerged in this study was how the study's student participants emphatically repeated the support by faculty for meaningful educational experiences as signally important. This study, which identifies the significance of supportive faculty to positive educational outcomes, supports the results of earlier studies.[16–18]

Along with faculty, family care and support was viewed as an important component of beneficial outcomes, such as retention and graduation from the program. Religion and spiritual beliefs were identified as integral to all aspects of life, including education. Students in this second study identified all these findings as imperative for positive educational experiences to take place.

Students clearly articulated their belief and views that health and illness were holistic concepts that could not be separated from religious beliefs. In this study, as in the first, students were uncomfortable with some of the teaching techniques and strategies used by faculty when teaching health and illness content in the curriculum and felt that there was a disparity in the educational material regarding what was taught about minority populations.

In this study, social interactions, viewed as important cultural expectations, were minimized while in the nursing program, which caused conflict with students and their family. Financial obligations for school and family life and the resources to meet these obligations varied among the students in this study, with few students receiving grants and scholarships and many working full time. Personal resources were developed that met the needs of their life ways and schedules, whereas college resources were underused by most students. All students described the importance of taking care of oneself, although, at the same time, acknowledging that they did not care for themselves well while in nursing school. A few of the ways they described lack of care of themselves were eating poorly, not exercising, not getting enough sleep, eating junk food for meals, snacking on junk food constantly while studying, not having time to get their hair cut, and no longer taking care of their fingernails or toenails. Students identified their lack of involvement and interest in political activities as a result of their other daily life demands.

As state earlier, a sincere desire on the part of the nurse educator to see the academic environment from a different perspective is a first key step to accommodation or negotiation to provide culturally congruent education to a diverse population of nursing students. Given that cultural care patterns are constantly changing, educators need to be willing to accept the notion that cultural diversity is a fact in the classroom and in the clinical environment with students. Thus, the path to culturally meaningful educational experiences begins with the nurse educators' sincere desire to provide culturally congruent education.

Discussions regarding best practices in nursing care become more evident each day. The implementation of nursing care moves toward evidence-based practice and best practices in all aspects of the nursing profession. These studies found that nurse educators not only need to teach students how to provide and practice in a culturally aware and congruent environment but that they must teach the art and science of nursing in the same way, by using evidence provided from research.

The literature also suggests that health care provided by caregivers from the same cultural, ethnic, and racial background as their patients usually provides more congruent health care experiences and better health care outcomes. Yet, minority nurses practicing today represent less than half the percentage of minorities in the general population. This disparity in numbers needs to be addressed and resolved. Finding ways to maintain minority students in nursing programs, to decrease attrition rates, and to recruit minority students all need to become a priority for the nursing profession. Studies like this one, a study that provides a better understanding of the cultural beliefs, values, and life ways of minority students, are a start on the path to resolution.

This study generally supports the findings of existing studies of African-American baccalaureate nursing students in predominantly white programs, but it deviates in one noteworthy aspect. Existing literature suggests that such nursing students feel that the institutional culture and environment do not match their own cultural heritage.[19] All students in this second study, however, responded that they were comfortable in their colleges and that the environmental context of the associate degree program did not pose a significant conflict. In addition, this study supports the few associate degree program studies that have been conducted, with African-American students identifying job conflicts, family responsibilities, and difficulty with time and scheduling.[20–22]

These findings have a significant implication for nursing faculty. The knowledge gained from these studies strongly suggests that thoughtful nursing educators need to find new ways to incorporate the care; understanding; and patience of family, friends, and faculty into teaching plans and processes they now use for the benefit of African-American students. Wider dissemination of the themes of these studies can assist nurse educators positively in the development of new nursing curricula that meet the values, beliefs, and practices of a diverse student body coming from a broadly diverse general populace. Nurse educators can begin to identify culturally congruent educational practices in the classroom and in clinical areas that enhance and support a more diverse student population. New and unusual teaching strategies that meet the educational learning styles of a more diverse student nurse population need to be identified, developed, and implemented.

These studies support the conclusion that students are more engaged and motivated to succeed if they know that faculty, family, and peers support them. Positive student-faculty relationships and a perception that the institution and nursing program are interested in their academic success can provide students with this crucial support. Although faculty members are plainly instrumental in initiating these relationships, students likewise bear individual responsibility to work toward establishing and nurturing these relationships.

SUMMARY

These two studies support and expand the existing literature on the importance of faculty, family, religion, and financial support for minority associate degree and baccalaureate degree nursing students. Although the second study with associate degree nursing students did not find the same strong sense of perceived unequal treatment as the first study with baccalaureate students, the associate degree study clearly articulated the same disparate educational expectations about education on minority population health assessment and nursing care. In addition, the recurring themes of overwhelming daily schedules and lack of college resources used to support student success provide nurse administrators and educators with important information that can assist colleges and schools of nursing with decisions about student scholarships and grant funding in the development of future college resources and programs.

Improving the number of graduating African-American nursing students has the potential to advance workforce diversity. Minority students who graduate from nursing programs and who then seek advanced degrees to educate future nurses contribute twofold: improving diversity among nurse educators and providing minority students with more and important ethnic role models within the nursing profession.

REFERENCES

1. US Department of Health and Human Services. Preliminary findings 2004 national sample survey of registered nurses. Available at: http://bhpr.hrsa.gov/healthworkforce/reports/rnpopulation/preliminaryfindings.htm. 2004. Accessed May 27, 2006.
2. Sullivan Commission. Missing persons: minorities in the health professions. Available at: http://www.kaisernetwork.org/health_cast/hcast_index.cfm?display=detail&hc=1141. 2004. Accessed June 30, 2006.
3. France N, Fields A, Garth K. "You're just shoved to the corner." The lived experience of black nursing students being isolated and discounted: a pilot study. Visions 2004;12:28–36.
4. Kosowski M, Grams K, Taylor G, et al. They took the time...they started to care: stories of African-American nursing students in intercultural caring groups. ANS Adv Nurs Sci 2001;23:11–27.
5. Gardner J. A successful minority retention project. J Nurs Educ 2005;44:566–8.

6. Tucker-Allen S, Long EG. Recruitment and retention of minority nursing students: stories of success. Lisle (IL): Tucker; 1999.
7. Labunski A. Addressing educational racism. J Nurs Educ 2003;11:2:481 [Electronic Version]. Available at: http://ut.ovid.com/gwl/ovidweb.cgi. Accessed June 15, 2006.
8. Barbee E, Gibson S. Our dismal progress: the recruitment of non-whites into nursing. J Nurs Educ 2001;40:243–4.
9. Childs G, Jones R, Nugent K, et al. Retention of African-American students in baccalaureate nursing programs: are we doing enough? J Prof Nurs 2004;20: 129–33.
10. Amaro D, Abriam-Yago K, Yoder M. Perceived barriers for ethnically diverse students in nursing programs. J Nurs Educ 2006;45:247–54.
11. Hassouneh D. Anti-racist pedagogy: challenges faced by faculty of color in predominantly white schools of nursing. J Nurs Educ 2006;45:255–62.
12. Aikens L, Cervero R, Johnson-Bailey J. Black women in nursing education completion programs: issues affecting participation. Adult Educ Q 2001;51: 306–21.
13. McQueen L, Zimmerman L. The role of historically black colleges and universities in the inclusion and education of Hispanic nursing students. ABNF J 2004;51–4 May/June.
14. Mills-Wisneski S. Minority students' perceptions concerning the presence of minority faculty: inquiry and discussion. J Multicult Nurs Health 2005;11:49–55.
15. Yoder M. The bridging approach: effective strategies for teaching ethnically diverse nursing students. J Transcult Nurs 2001;12:319–25.
16. Buckley J. Faculty commitment to retention and recruitment of black students. Nurs Outlook 1980;28:46–50.
17. Kersey-Matusiak GM. Black students' perceptions of factors related to their academic and social success in a predominately white undergraduate nursing program at a private Catholic college [Doctoral dissertation, Temple University, 1999]. Dissertation Abstracts International, DAI-A 60/7, 2370. 1999.
18. Elling TW, Furr SR. African American student in a predominantly white university: factors associated with retention. Coll Stud J 2002;36:188.
19. Wynetta LY. Striving toward effective retention: the effect of race on mentoring African American students. Peabody J Educ 1999;74:27–44.
20. Butters CR (2003). Associate degree nursing students. A study of retention in the nursing education program. [Doctoral dissertation, University of Massachusetts Boston, 2003]. Dissertation Abstracts International, DAI-B 64/10, 4862.
21. Hunt LB. A study of student retention in associate degree nursing programs as perceived by their directors [Doctoral dissertation, Ohio University, 1992]. Dissertation Abstracts International, DAI-A 53/10, 3453. 1992.
22. Sims GP. The experience of becoming a nurse: a phenomenological study of black women's experiences at predominantly white schools of nursing. [Doctoral dissertation, Georgia State University, 1996]. Dissertation Abstracts International, DAI-B 57/03, 1715. 1996.

Patient Education and Health Literacy

Katherine M. Zulick, BA[a],*, P. Alan Zulick, BA, JD[b],
Jane C. Rothrock, DNSc, RN, CNOR, FAAN[c]

KEYWORDS

- Health literacy • Patient education • English proficiency
- Communication • Language

A poor situation continues to worsen in the United States. Compared with other developed countries, the United States today has the largest annual health expenditures while Americans' life expectancy ranks the lowest. Not only do total dollar expenditures remain a genuine economic and political concern but they also represent a significant quality-of-life issue.

What contributes to the huge discrepancy between resources invested and quality of health outcomes? Scholars working on this question have come up with a surprising conclusion: one major contributing factor to poor health outcomes is inadequate health literacy.

HEALTH LITERACY DEFINED

What is health literacy? Ratzan and Parker offered an operational definition of health literacy. They viewed health literacy as "the degree to which individuals have the capacity to obtain, process, and understand basic health information and services needed to make appropriate health decisions."[1] Nielsen-Bohlman and colleagues[1] stated that nearly 50% of all American adults (almost 90 million out of 180 million people) have notable difficulty understanding and acting on health information. This percentage of people who have low levels of functional health literacy and the relative inability to translate literacy into successful negotiation of health information increases with age. When using Ratzan and Parker's operational definition—the ability to understand and act on health information to negotiate successfully to a positive health outcome—it is likewise important to define how one measures health literacy.

MEASURING HEALTH LITERACY: THE RAPID ESTIMATE OF ADULT LITERACY IN MEDICINE TOOL

There are a several approaches to measuring health literacy, one of which is the Rapid Estimate of Adult Literacy in Medicine (REALM). The REALM assessment tool uses

[a] Mount Holyoke College, South Hadley, MA, USA
[b] Pennsylvania Bar Association, Trial and Administrative Disciplinary Law, Media, PA, USA
[c] Perioperative Programs, Delaware County Community College, Media, PA, USA
* Corresponding author. 309 Washington Street, #3313, Conshohocken, PA 19428.
E-mail address: kmzulick@yahoo.com (K.M. Zulick)

Perioperative Nursing Clinics 4 (2009) 131–139
doi:10.1016/j.cpen.2009.02.001
1556-7931/09/$ – see front matter © 2009 Published by Elsevier Inc.

periopnursing.theclinics.com

a simple medical word recognition and pronunciation test to screen the adult patient's reading ability in medical settings. Staff who have minimal training can administer and score the test in less than 3 minutes, which makes it easy to use in clinical settings. Patients read from a list of 66 common medical terms that patients may encounter in their daily negotiation of personal health care. The medical terms are arranged in three columns according to the number of syllables and pronunciation difficulty. Thus, in column 1 (single syllable, easy to pronounce) might be the word "pill." The second column contains words with more syllables, which are more difficult to pronounce. This list might contain words such as "notify," "prescription," and "exercise." The final column contains the most difficult words; for example, "anemia," "diagnosis," and "osteoporosis." Each correctly read and pronounced word increases the test taker's score by one word or point. Scores can then be translated into four reading levels, based on grade level: grades 0–3 (0–18 words), grades 4–6 (19–44 words), grades 7–8 (45–60 words), and grade 9 and above (61–66 words).

To date, researchers have developed the REALM scale only in English, which creates obvious problems for its use within rising Spanish-speaking United States population groups or with other non-English speaking American patients. Furthermore, any scale developed in Spanish (and in similarly phonetic languages) necessarily would not be as valid because pronunciation measures would tend to fail, given the more straightforward linguistic structure of the Spanish language. In the Spanish language, there is usually a one-to-one correspondence between letters and sounds, making it somewhat easier to pronounce unfamiliar words, even for readers with limited health literacy skills.[1]

Another consideration with the REALM assessment test is that words used to gauge health literacy are not often taught in schools, which necessarily worsens the ability to use and process these words in personal health interactions. Unless one has had a reason to come into contact with some of the words (eg, "anemia" or "osteoporosis"), there is a good chance the average person in the United States will have trouble simply pronouncing those words. Conversely, how accurately one pronounces words may or may not equate to understanding those same words. One may be able to pronounce all 66 words, but still not know everything necessary about them to make appropriate medical decisions. Accordingly, the inferences one draws from REALM testing remain limited.

IMPACT OF HEALTH LITERACY

Today, one is hard pressed to go a single day without having to use one's health literacy. Whether reading pill bottles, calculating correct amounts of over-the-counter drugs, understanding medical brochures, following signs in medical settings, or deciphering online medical information, high health literacy demands pervade American society. A situation in which a patient is labeled as "noncompliant" may actually be a case of relative health illiteracy, which can occur in a patient who has low literacy skills and in one who has advanced literacy skills. People who have limited health literacy often lack knowledge or have misinformation about the body or the nature and causes of disease. Without this knowledge, they simply do not understand the relationship between what some perceive as simple lifestyle modifications, such as diet and exercise, and improving various health outcomes. Health information can overwhelm even persons who have advanced literacy skills. The science of medicine and surgery has progressed at an astounding pace. What a highly literate person learned during their school years quickly becomes outdated. An English professor, who possesses advanced literacy skills, may not recall information from a biology course. Health literacy strategies, such as using plain language, are as important for the literate patient as they are for the patient who has low literacy. Moreover, health information provided in a stressful or unfamiliar situation is unlikely to be retained. Thus, the need for comprehensive patient education strategies becomes compelling. The Joint Commission's "Understanding Your Caregivers" (**Fig. 1**), part of the Speak Up Campaign, offers questions that patients may have and provides answers to help patients understand the care they are receiving.

PATIENT EDUCATION MATERIALS

Information provided to patients can be overwhelming. They may find even the simple task of putting in one location all their medical information on one subject, such as an

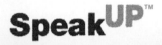

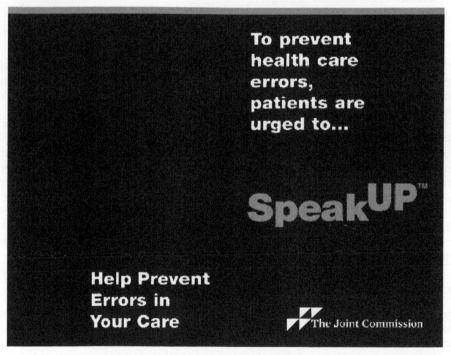

Fig. 1. "Understanding Your Caregivers" document. Available at: www.jointcommision.org/PatientSafety/SpeakUp/sp_understanding.htm. (*Courtesy of* The Joint Commission, Oakbrook Terrace, IL. © The Joint Commission, 2009. Reprinted with permission.)

upcoming surgery, too much to accomplish after merely getting through the day. Doing something as simple as providing a folder in which to keep all relevant medical information in one place can make a significant and positive difference in the patient's ability to logically process information and to prepare for what needs to be done in the order in which it needs to be done.

It is not uncommon at preoperative appointments for facilities to routinely provide a folder of important information on surgical procedures. Patients are also encouraged to keep any other relevant nonmedical information on that particular process in the same folder. In such folders, there is often a patient and family education booklet. In one specifically for lumbar spinal fusions, a table of contents may have headings such as the following:

Your spine
What is lumbar fusion surgery?
Reasons for fusion surgery
Potential complications of surgery
Preparing for surgery
What to expect in the hospital after the surgery
Discharge instructions

Sections for important phone numbers, patient and family notes, and questions may also be included. Although these sections are usually generic in their formatting, they include instructions to consult the physician for information specific to individual care and give the patient and family a good idea of what to expect.

Most daily physician–patient interactions, however, are for routine reasons, and initiatives in patient education must take this into account. Launched in 2001, the Joint Commission created its Public Policy Initiative aimed at addressing issues that could potentially compromise safe, high-quality care and the health of patients in the United States.[2] The Joint Commission initiative named three main policy objectives. First, it suggested that effective communications should be made an organizational priority to protect the safety of the patient. Next, it advised that health care provider–patient interactions should incorporate strategies to address patients' communication needs across the care continuum. Last, it determined that promotion of policy changes should be pursued to improve practitioner–patient communications.[2]

PATIENT EDUCATION AND INFORMED CONSENT

By 2007, The Joint Commission had published its report, "Hospitals, Language and Culture: a Snapshot of the Nation."[3] Recognizing the increasingly diverse patient populations served by the country's health care institutions, the qualitative cross-sectional study (the "snapshot") focused on answering questions about challenges and promising practices in serving culturally and linguistically diverse patients. Of the six research domains in the study, of significance to perioperative nurses was the domain of patient safety and provision of care. Although the recommendations and observations noted for all of the study domains were important, the data analysis revealed an area of particular significance and importance to patient safety: informed consent.

Determining whether the consent is on the patient's medical record is part of preoperative verification processes used by nurses in all perioperative procedure settings. Rothrock[4] noted that informed consent requires the health professional (in the case of surgery, the surgeon) not only to obtain the surgical consent but also to engage in a meaningful exchange of information and discussion with the patient. The legal interpretation of consent originates in the concept of battery (Appendix 1). Inherent in the concept of informed consent is the notion that an opportunity will be provided for a discussion and exchange of information. In the case of surgery, the discussion usually includes the type of surgery/name of the procedure, its risks and benefits, and reasonable alternatives. After such discussion, the patient signs the consent form, the signature is witnessed, the form is placed on the medical record, and its proper execution is noted before the start of surgery. What if, however, the form is in English and the patient and their family or significant others do not read or speak English?

Thus, the Joint Commission, in its report, "Hospitals, Language and Culture: a Snapshot of the Nation"[3] recommended that there should be formal processes for translating documents such as informed consent documents into languages other than English. They also recommended that health care interpreters be used during all informed consent processes when patients have limited English proficiency and that cultural brokers be used when the patient's cultural beliefs may impact the care proposed.

In the fall of 2008, the Joint Commission announced plans to use a grant from the Commonwealth Fund to develop accreditation standards for culturally competent, patient-centered care. These standards are targeted to take effect in 2011.[5] These standards will embrace health literacy as part of a broad definition of cultural competency as described by the National Quality Forum.[6] Effective communication with patients and the delivery of safe, equitable, and quality care are underpinned by issues of responding to diversity, culture, language, and health literacy.

IMPROVING PATIENT EDUCATION

Awareness, implementation, and constant improvement of communication strategies are paramount to improving health literacy. The Joint Commission charged medical practitioners with the following eight tasks: (1) to raise awareness of the impact of health literacy and English proficiency; (2) to train staff to recognize and respond appropriately to patients who have literacy and language needs so as to comply with the Joint Commission's National Patient Safety Goals; (3) to create patient-centered environments and to use clear communications in all interactions; (4) to use well-trained medical interpreters effectively for patients who have low English proficiency while providing reimbursement for their use; (5) to evaluate an organization's patient safety culture regularly, using valid and reliable tools such as the Agency for Healthcare Research and Quality hospital survey[7]; (6) to be aware of the practitioner's particular community, its literacy levels, and its language needs; (7) to make cultural competence a priority through hiring practices that value diversity and continuing education of staff; and (8) to continue to explore the impact of communication issues on patient safety, on disparities in health care, and on access to care.[2] Commins[8] offered an insightful discussion of one hospital's awareness of its particular community. Located in Arizona, it has a large Native American population. The hospital has made accommodations for the traditions of the Native Americans who live on a nearby reservation by building a nearby hogan for healing ceremonies and allowing the tribe's medicine man to come and pray over the patient. Clearly, cultural competence is a priority in this institution that understands how intimidating being admitted to a hospital can be for those who have different cultural beliefs.

PROVIDER–PATIENT ENCOUNTERS

Visits to a health care provider can feel overwhelming to any patient, not just those who have differing cultural beliefs. Smoothing the transition into the health care system should include eliminating "barriers to entry" by educating patients about when and where to seek care. A substantial amount of time and resources can be saved in the short-and long-term when patients use health services appropriately. Insurance enrollment forms, benefits explanations, and other insurance-related information should be developed into and provided in plain language that can be understood by patients who have limited health literacy. An appropriate literacy level should be considered when constructing this information; Seifert[9] noted that in general, these educational materials should be written at the fifth- or sixth-grade reading level.

Ensuring easy access to health care services can make an otherwise frustrating trip to the health care provider's office less stressful. Health care providers can assure such access with the use of clear, simple communications and signage, including the use of universal depictions combined with easy to understand descriptions.

Effective health care communication and educational materials need to be devised in alignment with three levels: literacy level, language, and cultural context. For example, directions to the local health clinic in a predominately poor community with limited health literacy might include very specific information about which bus line to take and where to find the bus schedule (all done in the appropriate language) in addition to the hours and contact information of that clinic. Depending on the community, potential patients may not have any means of private transportation.

The health care encounter itself can also be improved. Providers need to reinforce the use of plain language that is stripped of medical jargon and acronyms and not make assumptions about a patient's health literacy or education background. It is also important to avoid talking down to a patient. Making it clear that it is the standard policy to explain things in plain terms may help while one is getting to know a particular patient and his or her health literacy level, but the approach can be tailored as the provider–patient relationship grows. Tell-back collaborative inquiry or show-back techniques are essential to assess and ensure patient understanding, as is limiting information to two or three important points at one time and using drawings, models, or devices to demonstrate points.[10]

POLICY CHANGES THAT PROMOTE IMPROVED COMMUNICATIONS

Many of the solutions to improve provider–patient communications involve directly improving patient health literacy. Providers can consider tactfully referring patients who have low literacy to adult learning centers and assisting them with enrollment procedures. Within adult learning centers, a conscious move to develop and include health-related curricula is crucial to complement any policy changes within health care settings. Reimbursement policies for patient education must be broadened beyond diabetes to include other diseases and chronic conditions, because economics often plays a prominent, if unacceptable, role in health care education.

Making improved provider–patient communications economically appealing for those involved presents a bigger, more complex challenge. A potential path to instituting reimbursement policies for patient education involves pursuing pay-for-performance strategies that provide financial incentives and encourage patient-centered communications and culturally competent care. Practitioners have to be the first level of reform in patient education; an expansion in the number of medical liability insurance companies providing premium discounts to offices that receive education and training in patient-centered communications would go a long way toward more effective patient education. Conversely, increased premiums for those offices that do not participate in such training programs would facilitate transition to a more standard, national level of patient education. The expansion of the development of patient-centered educational materials and programs to support the increase of informed health care consumers is a sound investment for all.

SUMMARY

The United States health care system is at a crossroads. As countries worldwide struggle to find the best system for patients, providers, and health insurers, countries will increasingly begin to differentiate from each other vis-à-vis quality of health care. If the United States wants to provide the highest-quality health care to its people, it must first narrow and ultimately find ways to overcome the communication gap between those who have low health literacy levels or low English proficiency levels and the level of health literacy required to navigate the health care system. Processes that address language, culture, and health literacy promote shared decision making and informed choices. Forms and other written materials need to be translated. Other patient education enhancements such as videos and Web-based programs need to be made available in languages other than English. If America's health care providers truly believe in the concept of "choice" about which treatment path patients may choose based on their knowledge, preferences, and values, then health care providers must begin to use tools that objectively inform patients of their alternatives — while clarifying their preferences and values — and incorporate the patients' and the health care providers' perspectives in the decision making process. This is patient-centered care.

The changes suggested here are not only practical ways to improve the quality of health care for all Americans but are also sound economic proposals that in the end will promote the well-being of patients, providers, and even insurers if these initiatives are actively and fully pursued.

APPENDIX 1: LEGAL BRIEFS: HEALTH LITERACY AND INFORMED CONSENT

Health care professionals — physicians, surgeons, anesthesia providers, nurses, surgical technologists, and others in and out of hospitals — all want what is right for the patient and go to great lengths to make it happen. They routinely pay great attention to studying and enhancing things like patient health literacy, not just because they have to do so, but more often because they want to do so.[11,12]

Yet those same professionals also know it happens: a patient thinks he or she suffered an injury at their hands and sues, seeking monetary compensation. One possible cause of action that may arise, along with more usual claims of negligence-based malpractice, is the separate allegation of lack of informed consent.

Avoiding, minimizing, or managing such claims depends in large part on the entire team of health care professionals striving to assure that every surgical patient enjoys some more-than-minimum measure of health literacy. In the end, however, it is the surgeon's duty to assure that his or her patient amply demonstrates, orally and in writing, on a form and in the record, an informed consent so that the patient is empowered to say "yes" in a meaningful way to the surgical procedure about to happen.

Recent Pennsylvania case law and statutes illustrate how state jurists and legislators there have chosen to treat the action for lack of informed consent. In a 2002 case, the Pennsylvania Supreme Court addressed a separate claim of lack of informed consent, one that arose (as usually happens) in the context of surgery.[13] The court elaborated on informed consent this way [emphasis added]:

In a claim alleging lack of informed consent, it is the conduct of the unauthorized procedure that constitutes the tort.... A claim of a lack of informed consent sounds in the intentional tort of battery because an operation performed without the patient's consent is deemed to be the equivalent to a technical assault.... To obtain a patient's informed consent, doctors must provide patients with "material information necessary to determine whether to proceed with the surgical or operative procedure or to remain in the present condition."...This information must give the patient "a true understanding of the nature of the operation to be performed, the seriousness of it, the organs of the body involved, the disease or incapacity sought to be cured, and the possible results."...*While doctors are not required to disclose "all known information," they are required to "advise the patient of those material facts, risks, complications and alternatives to surgery that a reasonable person in the patient's situation would consider significant in deciding whether to have the operation." (p. 551, 1237)*

In addition to common law judicial construction, Pennsylvania, like other states, has now codified a controlling and expansive statutory version of informed consent requirements in its Health Care Services Malpractice Act,[14] as amended. Under that statute, except in emergencies, a physician owes a duty to the patient "to obtain the informed consent of the patient or the patient's authorized representative prior to conducting the following procedures: (1) Performing surgery, including the related administration of anesthesia...."[14]

Further, under the statute, the physician must provide the patient with a description of the procedure proposed, the risks and alternatives "that a reasonably prudent patient would require to make an informed decision...."[14] The statute also requires that in court cases, parties must offer expert testimony as to what constitutes informed consent, thus making bare assertions of informed and uninformed consent insufficient. Last, the jury may find the physician liable for failure to obtain informed consent "only if the patient proves that receiving such information would have been a substantial factor in the patient's decision...."[14] That is, showing a lack of informed consent will not suffice to justify an award unless the jury is persuaded that a reasonable person would have declined to proceed with the procedure if consent had been properly informed.

Researchers rightly continue to pursue ways to improve patient health literacy and better means and methods by which surgeons and health care professionals can secure informed consent.[15] These subjects are those that researchers need to pursue diligently. Additional reference to the body of state and federal law of informed consent remains a necessary adjunct consideration to that research.

REFERENCES

1. Ratzan SC, Parker RM. Introduction. In: Selden CR, Zorn M, Ratzan SC, et al, editors. National library of medicine current bibliographies in medicine: health literacy; 2000. Bethesda, MD: National Institutes of Health, U.S. Department of Health and Human Services. Cited in Nielsen-Bohlman L, Panzer A, Kindig D. Health literacy: a prescription to end confusion. Washington, DC: National Academies Press; 2004. p. 1, 32, 48.
2. The Joint Commission Public Policy Initiative. What did the doctor say? Improving health literacy to protect patient safety. Terrace (IL): The Joint Commission; 2007. p. 6–47.
3. Wilson-Stronks A, Galvez E. Hospitals, language and culture: a snapshot of the nation. The Joint Commission and the California Endowment. Chicago: The Joint Commission; 2007.
4. Rothrock JC. Can a nurse witness a surgical consent form before the anesthetist has seen the patient? Medscape nursing, ask the expert. Available at: www.medscape.com/viewarticle/488418. Accessed January 1, 2009.

5. The Joint Commission to Develop Hospital standards for culturally competent patient-centered care. Joint Commission Online. Available at: http://www.jointcommission.org:80/Library/jconline_sept_2008.htm. September 2008. Accessed September 18, 2008.
6. National Voluntary Consensus Standards for a Framework and Preferred Practices for Measuring and Reporting Cultural Competence. The National Quality Forum. Available at: www.qualityforum.org/projects/ongoing/cultural-comp/txReportVotingDraft%2011-19-08.pdf. Accessed January 19, 2009.
7. AHRQ: user's guide—hospital survey on patient safety culture. Available at: www.ahrq.gov/qual/hospculture/usergd.htm. Accessed December 2, 2008.
8. Commins J. Native Americans provide lesson in patient-centered care. Available at: www.healthleadersmedia.com/content/225214/topic/WS_HLMZ_COM/Nativ. HealthLeaders Media. Accessed December 17, 2008.
9. Seifert PC. Summer reading. AORN J 2008;88(2):177–8.
10. Kemp EC, Floyd MR, McCord-Duncan E, et al. Patients prefer the method of "tell back-collaborative inquiry" to assess understanding of medical information. J Am Board Fam Med 2008;21(1):24–30.
11. Lorenzen B. Using principles of health literacy to enhance the informed consent process. AORN J 2008;88(1):23.
12. Gates M. The 411 of informed consent. Radiology Today 2007;8(16):24.
13. Valles v Albert Einstein Med. Ctr. 569 Pa. 542, 551, 805 A.2d 1232, 1237 (2002).
14. Health Care Services Malpractice Act, 40 P.S. § 1303.504 (a), (b), (d), as amended.
15. Windle P. Understanding informed consent: significant and valuable information. J Perianesth Nurs 2008;23(6):430–3.

Educating Novice Perioperative Nurses

Beth Fitzgerald, RN, MSN, CNOR[a,b,c],*

KEYWORDS

- Educating nurses • Novice nurses
- Perioperative nurses education • Perioperative nursing
- Internship • Inservice training • Preceptorships

The first year for a perioperative novice nurse is filled with anxiety associated with their new role, the expectations of management and peers, and the realization of the tremendous responsibility entrusted to them by patients. At the Christiana Care Health System (CCHS), novice perioperative nurses have the opportunity to make the transition from novice to advanced beginner in a supportive environment where they can build their skills under the supervision and guidance of a qualified educator and dedicated preceptors. A perioperative internship program has been tailored to meet the needs of the facility and ensures novice nurses acquire a strong didactic and clinical foundation using evidence-based practices.

It is a well known fact that perioperative nursing is anticipating a nursing shortage crisis. Staff shortages continue to challenge operating room (OR) managers and directors, according to the *OR Manager* salary and career survey for 2008.[1] Training of novice nurses for the OR may take 8 months to 1 year depending on surgical specialties involved, and requires a significant investment of time and money. CCHS perioperative services have developed their own successful perioperative internship program to address the nursing shortage in its perioperative settings. This institution is financially and educationally committed to the customized program to support two inpatient and two outpatient surgery sites at two campuses, containing 56 ORs. The institution does not push the novice to begin practicing before they are ready and demonstrate competence. Training the novice perioperative nurse is viewed as an investment rather than a drain on resources.

THE CHRISTIANA CARE HEALTH SYSTEM PERIOPERATIVE INTERNSHIP PROGRAM

The CCHS Perioperative Internship Program is offered in collaboration with Delaware County Community College. The College offers 6 college credits and the hospital

[a] Christiana Care Health System, 625 W. 12th Street, P.O. Box 1668, Wilmington, DE 19899, USA
[b] Delaware County Community College, Media, PA, USA
[c] Perioperative Nursing, University of Delaware, Newark, DE 19716, USA
* Christiana Care Health System, 625 W. 12th Street, P.O. Box 1668, Wilmington, DE 19899
E-mail address: bfitzgerald@christianacare.org

Perioperative Nursing Clinics 4 (2009) 141–155
doi:10.1016/j.cpen.2009.01.006
1556-7931/09/$ – see front matter © 2009 Elsevier Inc. All rights reserved.

provides textbooks. This theory and evidence-based instruction provides the foundation for the novice perioperative nurse. The participants are provided copies of all policies, procedures, and clinical practice guidelines applicable to the OR. The novice nurse is encouraged to join Association of periOperative Registered Nurses (AORN) for support and additional educational material. They are also paid a registered nurse (RN) salary beginning on the first day of orientation.

The institution employs a full-time dedicated manager-educator to manage and teach the internship program. The educator must demonstrate a broad depth of perioperative clinical knowledge and excellent interpersonal skills. The educator prepares a syllabus (**Table 1**) with reading assignments; provides audiovisual materials, written examinations, and guest speakers; and teaches many of the classes. The educator is also responsible for managerial responsibilities, such as payroll, obtaining computer access, and so forth.

Selecting Candidates

Potential perioperative candidates are chosen by a rigorous selection process. New graduates are welcomed without medical or surgical experience; the well-known program attracts the best and brightest nursing students from local colleges and universities. The program accepts multigenerational learners from both the X and Y age bracket. Each candidate begins with an interview with human resources. The candidate is given an essay to complete: "Why I am a qualified candidate for the perioperative internship program." The candidate is asked to write this essay from their heart and include such information as communication skills, their ability to handle stress, realistic expectations of the job, and so forth. If the candidate has been approved by human resources, and the essay is of good quality, the candidate interviews with the internship program manager-educator.

This interview takes approximately 2 hours, because it involves the typical interview process, in addition to a detailed explanation of the program, expectations, and why working in the OR is not the glitz and glamour job that is depicted in the media. It is important to stress OR reality, dedication necessary for a perioperative career, and a perioperative passion. If the candidate meets the requirements, they are scheduled for a shadow day in the OR site of their choice. The shadow day consists of a tour of the OR by the site educator, followed by spending the day in an OR with staff nurses, then interviewing with the sites' interview team. The OR interview team determines if the candidate is acceptable. If the candidate accepts employment, they sign a 2.5-year contract to work at CCHS in the OR.

Program Overview

The Perioperative Internship Program at CCHS is offered in September and March, accepting 6 to 15 participants in each program, depending on staffing needs and budget constraints. The novice nurse spends their initial 12 weeks in a combination didactic, simulation laboratory, and clinical curriculum. The site for the didactic classroom presentations and simulation laboratory (**Fig. 1**) offers a conference room with audiovisual capabilities, a large storage room with a mock OR set up, and occasionally empty ORs for simulation practice. The classroom promotes a relaxed, stress-free environment. The chairs are comfortable, and attention to basic needs, such as snacks, frequent breaks, and room temperature, are supported.[2] This classroom is located near the ORs and simulation laboratory with the ability to move back and forth as needed for learning.

Required reading assignments accompany the classroom sessions. The goal of the course is to provide an introduction to perioperative nursing concepts and skills.

Theory, concepts, and evidence-based practice pertaining to both circulating and scrub roles are included. Course content is based on AORN's standards and recommended practices.

At the conclusion of the didactic, simulation laboratory, and clinical curriculum portion of the program, the novice enters phase II. During this time period, divided into 3-week blocks, the novice scrubs 5 days a week with a designated surgical technologist preceptor, following the preceptors' schedule, and learning one surgical specialty, such as neurosurgery, orthopedics, reconstructive surgery, and so forth. The next 3 weeks are spent with an RN preceptor in the circulating role, following the preceptors schedule and continuing in the same specialty for consistency. Ideally, the novice starts practicing in a simple general surgery specialty, but in reality the few general surgical cases necessitates the novice nurse start in the difficult neurosurgery or orthopedic specialties. This entire 6-week process of scrubbing and circulating is repeated in phase III in a different surgical specialty. The novice gains confidence in two surgical specialties after having established a rapport with the team members, repeated procedures, and constant reinforcement.

During phases II and III, the class meets once a month for roundtable discussions to share their experiences and war stories and continue the camaraderie that was formed in the classroom. The novice is able to ask questions in the safe environment of the classroom in addition to exploring reflective thinking, including "did I do that right?". This is an important time for the novice nurse as they compare experiences and begin to move to the advanced-beginner role. The novice needs to understand they are not alone in their quest for succeeding in the OR. Many novice perioperative nurses have high expectations and are often overachievers, expecting too much of themselves early in the didactic phase. They must constantly be informed that it takes at least 1 year for the novice to feel comfortable in the OR.

After successful completion of phase III, the novice then moves to the OR site cost center and continues their orientation by spending 2 to 3 weeks in each surgical specialty, 1 week scrubbing, and 1 to 2 weeks circulating until competent to perform independently. This process may take an additional 2 to 6 months depending on the OR site. This time period is spent with experienced surgical technologists and perioperative nurses to strengthen basic skills and develop service specialty skills. The novice becomes very anxious about moving to the new surgical specialties, because they have become comfortable and confident in the current specialty. As they move to the next surgical specialty rotation, especially an orthopedic or neurosurgery rotation, they fear moving to this new area requires higher expectations of their knowledge, performance, and skills. The novice is encouraged to observe the first day to build confidence. Higgins[3] has described this phase as a "trial run" because the novice is given the opportunity to expand their knowledge base, and apply it to new surgeries. The novice develops a gradual sense of insidership, increased self-esteem, and the ability to feel that they are participating in achieving their goals. The basic principle behind this phase is to ensure that newcomers can successfully demonstrate early successes in areas that are small enough be to achieved, but significant enough to excite enthusiasm.

Program Benefits

This perioperative internship program has eliminated the use of contract staffing at CCHS. The average cost of a contract nurse for 1 year is approximately $150,000. The cost for a perioperative intern without benefits is approximately $55,000 per year, a cost savings of $95,000 per year. This return on investment is well worth the effort of a hospital-based internship program. The expense is viewed as an investment

Table 1
Perioperative internship program syllabus for weeks 2 and 3

Day	Content	Faculty	Policies/CPGs	Assignment	Resources
Week 2: September 15, 2008					
Monday September 15, 7:30–4 RCA, Classroom/Lab	Class/Lab Day 3, Establishing sterile field, back table/ mayo/, draping demonstration, lab Continue SGG, G&G another, create sterile field	—	—	Aseptic technique quiz	Lab: Continue SGG, back table/mayo set up, Cloth and paper custom packs
Tuesday September 16, 7:30–4 RCA, Lab	Lab Day 4, Lab – Continue SGG, G&G another, create sterile field, instruments	—	—	Before today's class: Read: Alexander's Ch 6: pp 173–182; AORN's RPs: Instruments and powered equipment: care and cleaning	Video: basic OR instrumentation Video: care and handling of surgical instruments, instrument books
Wednesday September 17, 7:30–4 RCA, Classroom/Lab	Class Day/Lab Day 5, Suture (basic overview), counts/ incorrect count, sharps disposal, universal protocol/ FRA, Lab – Continue SGG, G&G another, create sterile field	—	P&P counts, P&P – sharps disposal, P&P correct site Sx.	Before today's class: Read: Alexander's Ch. 2 pp 27–31, pp 39–42 Also read AORN Guidance Statement on Sharps Injury Prevention & RP - Counts	Paper ID forms, CPG – Preoperative Care ID of patient, procedure, and universal protocol
Thursday September 18, 7:30–4 RCA, Classroom/Lab	Class/Lab Day 6, surgical conscience, Lab – create sterile field, loading, passing, counting, instruments/ needles/blades	—	—	UP quiz	—

Friday September 19, 7:30–4 RCA, Classroom/Lab	Class/Lab Day 7, compression boots, create sterile field, Foleys/counting, placing patient on OR bed, placing armboards	—	Nursing Procedures, 2.2–sequential, compression boots, Foley best practice, Foley policy	Before today's class: Read: AORN's RPs: Guidance Statement - Prevention of Venous Stasis	Continue set up back table, mayo, draping, loading, passing, hypos, counting, instruments/needles/blade, Video: Foley
Week 3: September 22, 2008					
Monday March 10, 7:30–4 RCA, Lab	Class/Lab Day 8, Lab - Loading, passing, counting, instruments/needles/blades, Continue circulating skills, Continue set up back table, mayo, draping, hypos	—	Map – COR, Notebook information, unit/facility, introduction	—	Compression boot practice, Foley, student/preceptor info, skills assessment completed, notebooks
Tuesday March 11, 7:00–3:30, clinical sites	Clinical Day 1, scrub, COR – scrub and observe only	Preceptors	—	—	—
Wednesday March 12, 7:00–3:30, clinical sites	Clinical Day 2, scrub	Preceptors	—	—	—
Thursday March 13, 7:00–3:30, clinical sites	Clinical Day 3, scrub	Preceptors	—	—	—
Friday March 14, 7:30–4 RCA, classroom	Class Day, back safety/body mechanics/needle sticks, variance reports, risk management, consent	Employee Health, Nurse, 10:00, LCD, Risk Management 1:00	P&P – needlestick injury, needlestick packet, CCHS policy, informed consent CCHS policy, event reporting CCHS policy, disclosure policy CCHS policy, sentinel events	Before today's class, reread: AORN Guidance statement: sharps injury prevention in the perioperative setting; creating a patient safety culture; the position statement Workplace safety; Alexander's, Ch 2, surgical consents, sentinel events, pp 27–31	Medcom Trainex, consent forms

Intern will bring competency to clinical: SG&G.

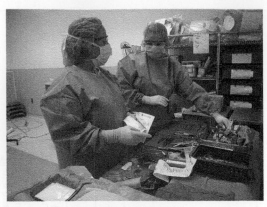

Fig. 1. Students practicing in the simulation laboratory.

in improving the quality, safety, and efficiency of care in the OR. A questionnaire is provided at the end of the 6-month program to evaluate the novice nurses' view of the program, and to assess the program's effectiveness (**Box 1**). With answers such as, "I feel more confident each day. When I do something new, I feel my knowledge increase. I am much less nervous now," it is evident the novice perioperative nurse education is effective. The novice perioperative nurse brings enthusiastic learners into the OR, informs veteran staff of changes in recommended practices, and provides safe patient care.

SELECTING THE NOVICE NEW GRADUATE

Concerns have been expressed in the literature regarding hiring new graduates in a novice perioperative program. Traditionally, many institutions believe new graduates are not appropriate in the OR, and require 1 year of medical or surgical experience before entering a perioperative educational program. There are many opinions regarding hiring new graduates versus the experienced nurse. Vahey states that 1 year on a medical-surgical unit is an excellent way for the graduate nurse to bridge nursing education with nursing practice, and to prepare for the health care environment. This medical-surgical experience builds an invaluable foundation for future practice.[4] Lund disputes the need for a 1-year medical-surgical experience, stating there is no evidence to support or refute the premise that new graduates should work in medical-surgical nursing before working in a specialty area.[4] A perioperative program can be designed for all graduate nurses and RNs, regardless of experience level. Experienced RNs from other fields can be excellent candidates for a perioperative program because they usually have the ability to organize and prioritize. Graduate nurses are also good candidates because they are still in a learning mode, and tend to absorb material rapidly and are not afraid to question the educator. An RN with more education and experience is not necessarily a better nurse than a peer who has less education or experience.[5]

Another concern is failure to pass the NCLEX. If the novice is unable to pass the NCLEX, they are able to remain in the perioperative program, but function in the scrub role with a surgical technologist preceptor until they pass the NCLEX. The hourly wage is decreased by half, but the novice is able to continue with the classroom work and assignments. After passing the examination, the novice resumes the circulating role and completes the circulating competencies. This route may take the novice nurse

Box 1
Graduating class questionnaire

1. How did you feel on your very first day in the internship class?

Nervous.

I was nervous because I wasn't sure of what to expect, but after the first hour I was fine because it is a very relaxed atmosphere to learn.

I was very excited to meet my fellow classmates and to start working toward my goal of becoming a perioperative nurse!

2. How did you feel during your first day in clinical?

Like I was going to pass out. Sacred to death I was going to mess something up.

I was nervous, excited and a little scared, but turned out to be a fantastic experience. I was not alone and helped along the way.

Overwhelmed with the size and scale of the OR.

I was very excited and scared at the same time, mostly because it was a whole new environment that I was not used to.

3. What helped you succeed during these past 6 months?

I feel the staff, from environmental staff to the physicians (most of them) were and are very friendly and supportive in making me feel welcomed, comfortable, and part of the family.

One or two certain people who were my preceptors, who cared about me right from the start when others brushed me off as "just another periop."

Determination to succeed in what I have been passionate about since starting my nursing career.

4. How do you feel today about working in the OR, the internship program, and your past 6 month experience?

I love working in the OR. The internship helped prepare me for this position. Sometimes I can't believe I am being paid for doing my job because I enjoy it so much!

Overall feeling is good. Bad days and good days. Frustrated at times, yet satisfied at times.

I've learned a great deal, not just about things like instruments and procedures, but about how staff interact with others and the different dynamics that occur within the OR team. I feel confident in many areas that I didn't think I would. Yet, there are still days that are incredibly frustrating.

longer to complete the perioperative program, but experience demonstrates graduates that have not passed the NCLEX the first, second, or third time have become very strong successful perioperative nurses.

THEORETICAL AND CONCEPTUAL FRAMEWORK

Many theoretical frameworks and models are used in a perioperative program. When teaching a perioperative novice class with many different generational, educational, and life experiences, adhering to one model or framework structure is inadequate. The most important framework used in a novice perioperative program is Benners'[6] theory described as "Novice to Expert." The novice has no experience of the situations or skills in the OR in which they are expected to perform; the novice must be taught the perioperative principles necessary for the skill development. The information must be taught to the novice in measurable and objective principles relating to the OR. Benner[6] describes the Dreyfus Model of Skill Acquisition as a student passes through the learning stages from novice to expert.[6] The Dreyfus model is a general guide and measures learner's proficiency levels. The novice has no perioperative experience, so they must be given a foundation and guiding principles to direct their performance, even though the guiding principles rules cannot tell the novice the most relevant tasks to perform in an actual or emergent situation.[6] Skilled performance is achieved through principles and theory learned in the classroom and the context-dependent judgments and skill are acquired as the novice moves into clinical rotations. The novice perioperative nurse is taught the tasks that take place in the OR without the situational experience.[6] The Dreyfus model states that beginners must operate on abstract principles, formal models, and theories to get into the situation in a way that they can learn safely and efficiently.[6]

Because of high numbers of older learners, Knowles' Principles of Adult Learning is used throughout the program. Knowles realized that adults learn in a manner different from that of children; the novice learns best when treated as an adult. The perioperative novice program requires the adult learner to assume responsibility for learning and the use of perioperative resources.[7]

Kolb's Model of Experiential Learning is used because it places less emphasis on educator-centered learning and more emphasis on the novices' use of experiences in the learning process. Novice knowledge is acquired by transforming experiences into new ways of thinking; learning is increased when students are actively engaged in gaining knowledge with experiential problem solving and decision making.[7] Kolb describes learning as a four-stage cycle, with learning occurring as a person cycles from concrete experience (feeling); to reflective observation (watching); to abstract conceptualization (thinking); to active experimentation (doing).[7] Reflective observation about the experience is essential to the learning process, because it links the concrete experience to abstract conceptualizations of the experience, allowing the novice to practice active experimentation.[7] At the beginning of the perioperative program, the novice relies on the abstract principles of didactic learning, but eventually uses concrete experience and moves toward active experimentation in the OR. The clinical learning takes place in the OR because experience is paramount for expertise. It is important for the novice to have experiences in the OR soon after completion of mastering a new concept because the best way for the novice to learn is with hands-on training. The novice grasps the new experience and then transforms the experience into new behaviors.[8] This model encourages the novice to use their critical thinking skills through reflection. The novice reflects on clinical experiences, evaluates what was done correctly, and notes opportunities for improvement. The novice then develops ideas on how to proceed, actively experiments with actions to test the ideas, and eventually develops competence through the experiences. The novice participates in experiential learning and in doing so acquires a degree of clinical competency over time.[8]

Blooms taxonomy is applied to the novice perioperative program. Because perioperative nursing is a practice discipline that ultimately requires the application and synthesis of acquired knowledge, skills, and attitudes, the educator must progress from the simple concepts to the complex. The underlying assumption is that each subsequent level builds on and integrates the prior set of knowledge, skills, and attitudes.[7] The order of presenting perioperative content assists the novice in becoming successful, and allows them to experience satisfaction and a sense of accomplishment. The perioperative novice has a lack of confidence; is afraid to make mistakes; and is scared, nervous, stressed, and very anxious. Teaching in a simple building block format decreases anxiety and allows the novice to learn. The curriculum is designed to provide the novice with a strong foundation of knowledge and experience before they enter the OR. The curriculum builds on the novice's existing skills, beginning with simple skills, such as infection control, and then working toward more complex skills, such as the surgical scrub-rub. After the basic technical elements of the surgical scrub are mastered, the novice is taught gowning and gloving. These skills are then integrated, return demonstrations are performed and perfected, and the novice progresses to learning aseptic technique. Focusing on one activity at a time promotes the novice nurses' success because the novice is able to practice the skill, gain competence in using and refining the skill, and continues to learn through return demonstration and reinforcement.

Competency-based education identifies the critical thinking skills, knowledge, technical skills, and attitudes novice nurses need to develop if they are to achieve program outcomes. Competencies are the behavioral, observable evidence of clinical knowledge. Competency assessment is an objective measurement of an individual's performance of essential job responsibilities. Competency is what a nurse is capable of doing, and it is manifested in measurable actions and behaviors.[9] Competency is a level of performance measured against professional standards, such as AORN; Joint Commission; the risk management department; and the institution's policies, procedures, and clinical practice guidelines. The novice must demonstrate their ability to perform perioperative skills and activities, and is responsible for their own learning. The educator becomes the facilitator, guiding the novice in achieving the competencies. Competencies allow the educator to assess and validate the novice nurse's skills. The competency can be developed in an easy-to-understand format, and after completion is placed in the novice nurse's permanent file. **Fig. 2** demonstrates a simple checklist competency that serves as a guide by which preceptors can evaluate specific technical skills. They are developed from the OR policies, procedures, and clinical practice guidelines. A surgical procedure checklist is used later in the novice's orientation as they move through each surgical specialty. The skills checklist helps the novice follow their own progress, and drives them to map out future learning needs. Competencies are used to identify knowledge gaps and skill deficits in a timely manner to customize a remediation plan.

TEACHING STRATEGIES

Each novice has a different learning style, and the educator must appeal to each of these styles. Unfortunately, there is no one teaching strategy that is effective for the entire class; learning strategies must be intertwined to respect the diverse methods of learning. The educator needs to incorporate a variety of teaching strategies while being creative, committed, stimulating, and motivating. The educator needs a sense of humor, and works many long overtime hours to create a successful program. The novice needs to trust the educators' perioperative expertise, knowledge of educational theory, evidence-based practice, and research. When teaching, the educator needs also to take a personal interest in the novice: being sensitive to their feelings and problems, expressing respect and concern for them, alleviating their anxieties, being accessible and available, being fair, allowing different points of view, creating an atmosphere in which they feel free to ask questions, and most importantly showing the novice nurse a sense of warmth and caring. On the first day of class, educational and clinical expectations should be clearly stated. Communicate high expectations because the novice is expected to work hard. The educators' excitement about the OR and sharing of clinical experiences also inspire the novice nurse to succeed.

PERIOPERATIVE COMPETENCY WORKSHEET

Competency: Performs Surgical Hand Scrub/Rub, Sterile Gowning and Gloving
Gowning and Gloving Another

Domain: Safety

Competency Statement: Performs surgical hand scrub according to procedure and observes
principles of aseptic technique before every operative procedure.

PERFORMANCE CRITERIA	METHOD OF EVALUATION RD, O, D, C	INITIALS

1. Complies with hospital policy regarding surgical attire.
    a. Hair and jewelry confined
    b. Scrub Shirt tucked in
    c. Protective eye wear in place
	RD,O	

2. Performs surgical hand scrub and rub according to procedure and manufactures directions.	RD, O	
3. Gowns self from separate table.	RD, O	
4. Dons sterile gloves using closed gloving method.	RD, O	
5. Wears two pairs of gloves (double gloves) – standard precautions.	RD, O	
6. Changes failed glove as promptly as patient safety permits.	RD, O	
7. Assists others with donning sterile gown and gloves.	RD, O	
8. Monitors sterility of team during surgery and takes corrective action as soon as possible.	RD, O, D	
9. Correctly removes gown and gloves without contamination.	RD, O	

Method of Evaluation Key: RD – Return Demonstration, O – Observation, D – discussion C – Chart
Review

PRECEPTOR SIGNATURE _____ DATE _____

Comments:

Plan for next week:

Opportunities for improvement:

Fig. 2. Perioperative competency worksheet.

The novice rises to meet the expectations if they are motivated and are given the
support and encouragement they need.

Lecturing can be an efficient and effective method of introducing learners to new
topics, although novices are passive listeners and tune out before the end of class
and miss important information. If the educator is a clinician working in the OR where
practice and technology is constantly changing, they are able to convey both the
content and the excitement of the OR through the lecture method. The educator is
the authority on the OR, a role model who has developed expertise in the field, shares
their knowledge, and understands theories of the novice learner. The lecture strategy
encourages students to develop listening abilities that are required in the OR. There
are disadvantages of lecturing. Teaching facts places little emphasis on problem
solving, decision making, and critical thinking.[10]

Lecturing can be combined with a show and tell strategy. Presenting dressings and
drains, their importance, and use in the OR is much more interactive if the educator
passes around the different dressings and drains used in the OR during the lecture.

The novice can touch, feel, and picture in their mind why a dressing is used on a special type of incision or wound.

The discussion strategy can be used after the lecture. The educator can give the novice class an opportunity to apply the principles, concepts, and theories discussed in the lecture. This clarifies misconceptions and allows the educator to observe if learning has occurred. This method is very effective with a small perioperative class. The disadvantage of the discussion strategy is time. Discussions can become very time consuming because the novice class excitedly relates their clinical experiences to the discussion. Many times discussions lose sight of the original thoughts, and the educator must keep the novice class focused on the discussion at hand.[10]

The questioning strategy has the educator asking questions to assess the novice nurses' comprehension and retention of information. The educator asks questions that test the novices' reasoning, analysis, and problem-solving skills. Asking questions that elicit critical thinking and content review demonstrates to the educator if the novice understood the information. A thoughtful question asked by the educator or the novice can create a lively discussion. The educator can also present a "what would you do if" and ask the class to come up with a solution.[10]

Audiovisual aids are excellent teaching strategies as long as the educator is careful not to use videos for time filler and entertainment. Pictures, charts, overhead transparencies, CD ROMs, DVDs, whiteboards, and computer programs are all useful to the perioperative program. Some aids, such as DVDs, are expensive, but one can create visual aids for very little cost. A heavy poster board composed of sterilization indicators can help the novice with different sterilization techniques and the different indicators and integrators. Audiovisual aids can also be incorporated into the lecture or discussion phase.[10]

Cooperative learning is a fun teaching strategy because the educator structures small groups that work together toward achieving a shared learning goal. The group is responsible not only for their own learning, but also for the other novice nurses in the group.[10] For example, the novice class is separated into groups of three. The groups are given strips of paper describing perioperative nursing responsibilities that need to be accomplished before a surgical case begins. The group places the strips in the order of how they would accomplish preparing for a generic surgical case. This promotes the role of a functioning team member. This actively also enhances social skills as the novice learns to communicate with their colleagues.

The simulation strategy is a controlled representation of reality as the novice learns about the real world without the risks of the real world. This is another fun strategy, because the novice practices psychomotor skills in a simulation laboratory controlled setting, and can apply the principles about which they have read.[10] Coordination of what is taught in class is then immediately practiced in laboratory. The technical aspects of the surgical environment are explored, and basic perioperative skills are practiced in the simulation laboratory. Demonstrations with return demonstrations of draping a patient, loading suture, and so forth are documented. The novice is able to start sequencing a surgical procedure, and pull together the skills they have practiced separately, such as gowning and gloving another, draping the patient, and so forth. This strategy is not only helpful for those performing the procedure, but the observers are able to learn and critique at the same time. Simulation is also used with role playing. The novice nurse can role play the part of a surgeon and patient to develop an understanding of what it is like on the "other side."

Supplies for the simulation laboratory require great effort on the part of the educator-manager. Every OR has surgical cases that have been cancelled. The opened, clean soft goods, such as custom packs, sponges, drapes, gowns, gloves, suture, can be saved by OR staff members. The supplies are collected by the educator and stored in the simulation laboratory (items that cannot be used are boxed and sent to third-world countries). This is a cost effective way to support the simulation laboratory.

Using case studies is an excellent way of analyzing an incident or situation in which an event has happened, and the problem needs to be solved.[10] The case study may focus on a poor outcome situation or never-event from the OR. After giving details of the incident, the novice learner responds to the question "What would you do?" This strategy initiates discussion and engages critical thinking skills.

Journaling each day is an underused method of uncovering novice difficulties and struggles. The novice may be instructed to document their experiences of the clinical day, how they felt about the experience, what new skill they learned, and any challenges encountered. The novice may reveal, in writing, challenges they do not feel comfortable expressing in class. Journals can be collected every week to track the novice's progress.

PRECEPTORS

Preceptors play the most important role in training the novice nurse, and are the key to a successful novice perioperative program. The educator cannot be in every OR every day; consequently, the preceptor must take over and continue the education of the novice. The preceptor guides the novice by showing them a procedure; allowing them to assist; then allowing them to practice independently, but with close supervision. This is why the role of the perioperative preceptor is so very important.

The qualifications of an effective preceptor are numerous. Preceptors need to be enthusiastic, willing and able to teach, and possess professional communication tools. The preceptor is a role model, conscientious, patient, kind, and knowledgeable. They must be a team player and able to collaborate with all the surgical team members. Learning takes place best in a nonthreatening environment; preceptor attitude and gestures can make or break a novice perioperative nurse. The preceptor creates a competent, confident perioperative nurse.[11] This is a tall order for a staff member successfully to fulfill. The preceptor needs to critique the novice at the end of each day, informing them of what was successful, opportunity for improvement, and future goals. The novice and preceptor also collaborate on next day surgical cases to meet the needs of the novice experience. Preceptors need much support and encouragement.

Appropriate selection and training of preceptors can guarantee success. Ideally, excellent preceptors have been through the same perioperative novice program. Preceptors follow AORN recommended practices and OR policies, procedures, and clinical practice guidelines.

The preceptors and educator need constant communication and collaborating. Rewarding and recognizing the preceptor with constantly saying "thank you," showing personal and work-oriented concern, and valuing their ideas and incentives are very important. Incentives, such as gift certificates to the cafeteria, movie tickets, or beach towels imprinted with the hospital logo, are inexpensive but much appreciated by the preceptor. Some institutions reward preceptors with $1 more per hour or offer spot bonuses. Incentives show the preceptor that the institution recognizes and values their extra role and effort.

Precepting can place a strain on staff because novice orientation is ongoing, and staff become worn out and weary and tire of the continual flow of novice nurses.

The preceptors tend to become overworked, and burn out. As a result, finding quali-fied preceptors can be difficult.

The preceptors should complete a perioperative preceptor program or workshop. This workshop should be organized and taught by the educator-manager, other perioperative educators, and surgical technologist, and RN preceptors.

MANAGER AND EDUCATOR ROLE IN PREPARING THE NOVICE

The perioperative novice nurse educator must possess a deep passion for the OR and the desire to teach and share knowledge, in addition to spending extra time and effort that is required for a successful perioperative program. The educator has a responsi-bility for the future of perioperative nursing, and to inform the novice of current National Safety Patient Goals and Joint Commission requirements. The educator provides education and training in a classroom and simulation laboratory setting and constantly needs to remember what it was like to be a perioperative novice. Much advanced preparation is needed because textbooks need to be ordered, policies and proce-dures need to be copied, a syllabus must be prepared, presentations and lectures organized, and guest speakers arranged. The simulation laboratory must be organized and supplies must be stored.

The manager side of this position is responsible for interviewing, hiring, completing hiring forms, payroll, and mentoring the novice perioperative nurses during the program. Preceptor schedules require confirmation to provide consistency to the novice nurse. The novice nurse is provided with the managers' beeper and office tele-phone numbers to ensure constant communication. The manager needs to caution the novice nurse regarding OR behavior. The novice wants to make a good impression and "be one of the OR nurses" and may step on toes or contaminate the atmosphere.

The manager-educator is an advocate of the novice, reducing frustration, assisting with staff interactions, and providing collegial and supportive leadership. The novice perioperative nurses all have the same concerns. The educator must listen, observe, and constantly assess the novice. Communication is the key to a successful program. The educator must consistently communicate with the novice to ensure the program is meeting their needs, and take time to work out problems or answer questions, allow-ing the novice to feel welcome and comfortable in the OR.

Daily clinical rounding by the educator is the ideal, but the reality is weekly or twice weekly rounds because the manager-educator may have other responsibilities to the perioperative department. Rounds are conducted to monitor the novice's progress, identify struggles, and give positive encouragement.

EVALUATIONS

Evaluation is an ongoing process that determines the novice's progress, promotes the professional growth of the novice, and improves the quality of the teaching-learning process.

Perioperative educators are accountable to the community to ensure the compe-tency of its nurses, and the evaluation of the novice nurse is a method to support this responsibility. Evaluation should occur throughout the orientation process with the learner and educator communicating constantly on progress, identifying strengths and opportunities for improvement, changes needed in the syllabus or methods of teaching, and assessing the effectiveness of the perioperative program.

There are many means of evaluation in a novice perioperative program. The perio-perative course and program and the educator must be evaluated by the novice nurse. The novice must evaluate themselves and their preceptors. Feedback from physicians, staff, site educators, and leadership staff is solicited for evaluations. Program retention rates are reviewed. The novice's learning is evaluated with written tests, quizzes, case studies, simulation laboratory return demonstration of skills, case logs, preceptor evaluations, review of clinical performance, and competency assessments. A written evaluation for each novice at the completion of the program identifies areas of strength, personal and professional growth and development, constructive feedback regarding accomplishments, desired changes in performance or behavior, and setting future measurable goals. Negative feedback must be given in a constructive manner, in a private place. Feedback should be specific and directed toward the act, not the person, and comparisons with other class members must be avoided. The manager needs to listen, express views, and encourage solutions. An evaluation questionnaire is also given to each novice nurse as they complete the perioperative program (see **Box 1**).

Course evaluations are effective communication tools, but not always reliable as a single measure of quality. After reviewing the course evaluation, the manager makes changes to improve, refine, and strengthen the program for the next class. For example, the novice perioperative program was originally designed to rotate scrubbing for 1 week, circulating for 1 week, and continue with this rotating process throughout the first 12 weeks. Novice feedback brought about a change in scrubbing for a consistent 4-week timeframe, and circulating for a consistent 4-week timeframe.

MANAGING THE STRUGGLING NOVICE

Occasionally, a novice does not succeed or is not the right fit. Frequent observation and communication with the novice is crucial if challenges are evident. The educator may notice the novice is not prepared in the classroom, has difficulty with return demonstrations in the simulation laboratory, or may not be able to comprehend the demands of the OR. Do not avoid these issues, because the problem may not resolve with time and they may never be a viable employee. Begin documentation of incidents, form a close relationship with human resources, and deal with the issues immediately and directly. Communicate with the novice and send a clear message regarding expectations along with a timeline, and then follow through if the expectations are not met. The disciplinary process should begin with a written statement containing specific facts and dates. The novice is not required to sign the statement. This document provides the novice with an opportunity to improve. During discussion with the struggling novice, discuss learning tools and activities, develop an action plan, and set realistic target dates for improvement. The action plan may include reviewing a total joint instrumentation set with an orthopedic-savvy nurse or a redemonstration with return demonstration. If there is no improvement within the time frame, and the goals are not met, the novice may be offered reassignment.

GRADUATION

A graduation ceremony is held for the novice perioperative nurse as they move into the advanced-beginner period. The graduation is held on the last day of the 12-week didactic, simulation laboratory, clinical program to celebrate successful completion of the perioperative program. A catered lunch is provided and certificates from the college are formally distributed. OR bouffant hats decorated with tassel ribbon are worn as the graduating class is photographed. Fear, uncertainly, and frustrations have decreased because of the foundation of knowledge and skill provided by the perioperative program. The novices have been supported by the educator-manager, and have also provided support to each other in the nonthreatening, safe, protected learning environment of the classroom. They have been presented with a sense of direction and do not fear abandonment at the conclusion of the didactic portion of the program. The novice perioperative nurse has learned how to implement safe perioperative care to their patients, and always remembers there is a patient who is not aware of interventions under the drapes. The novice now understands the problems that the patient brings to the surgical experience and recognizes the outcomes essential to intraoperative interventions.

SUMMARY

The emphasis of perioperative novice education is to prepare the novice nurse for the professional practice of perioperative nursing. Perioperative patient care is based on sound perioperative evidence-based practice and nursing principles, which enables the novice to plan patient care with greater confidence. Teaching novice perioperative nurses is both rewarding and laborious, but to see the novice perioperative nurse grow, gain confidence, and become a successful perioperative nurse who in 2 years attains the level of CNOR makes the effort worthwhile. Perioperative nursing is constantly changing and the educator-manager needs continually to devise and develop new ways of ensuring nurses are continually prepared for the future. Perioperative nurse educators have a commitment to the communities they serve to ensure high-quality, competent perioperative practice that emphasizes the delivery of safe perioperative patient care to patients. A solid novice perioperative education program integrating nursing theory and AORN standards provides the novice nurse with a strong foundation of knowledge in caring for the surgical patient.

REFERENCES

1. Saver C. Overtime, new grads help stretch staffing in hospital operating rooms. OR Manager 2008;24(9):1–11.
2. DeSilets L, Pinkerton S. Quality…I'll know it when I see it. J Contin Educ Nurs 2004;35(3):100–1.
3. Higgins J. Thinking outside the box: perioperative preceptorship. Can Oper Room Nurs J 2004;22(1):37–40.
4. Lund P, Vahey D. Should medical-surgical nursing experience be required for new graduates before working in a specialty? MCN Am J Matern Child Nurs 2005;30(3):160–1.
5. Geslak J. When resources are scarce, consider growing your own. AORN J 2005; 82(2):244–9.
6. Benner P. From novice to expert. New Jersey: Prentice Hall; 2001. p. 20–1.
7. Billings D, Halstead J. Teaching in nursing a guide for faculty. St. Louis (MO): Elsevier Saunders; 2005. p. 27, 28, 198, 215.
8. Sewchuk D. Experiential learning: a theoretical framework for perioperative education. AORN J 2005;81(6):1311–8.
9. Stobinski J. Perioperative nursing competency. AORN J 2008;88(3):417–36.
10. DeYoung S. Traditional teaching strategies. In: DeYoung S, editor. Teaching strategies for nurse educators. New Jersey: Prentice Hall; 2003. p. 113–44.
11. McNamara S. Teaching others the "why" of what we do. AORN J 2005;82(1):9–11.

Developing Simulation Scenarios for Perioperative Nursing Core Competencies and Patient Safety

Christine E. Smith, RN, MSN, CNOR

KEYWORDS

- Simulation • Scenarios • Perioperative • Competency
- Education • Patient safety

The perioperative environment, an interdisciplinary team–dependent care model within a highly complex, technologically dense, and human factor–reliant care system, provides rich opportunities to practice, test, investigate, and validate patient-care processes. The patient's risk for injury is great and errors can be made in every process and procedure in this environment. Active learning exercises in a clinically realistic setting can improve the acquisition of psychomotor performance, ability to think critically and make decisions, clinician confidence, professional satisfaction, and interpersonal team skills. Simulation scenario training is a valuable educational tool for the perioperative setting. Such training prepares clinicians, but also assists in meeting regulatory expectations and promotes patient and staff safety. Furthermore, such training is useful for experienced clinicians, but especially for clinicians entering the workplace for the first time. These health care providers bring with them new core social, interpersonal, technological, learning and lifestyle needs and values, and are especially responsive to the educational technique used with simulation scenario training.

Perioperative and interventional procedure services are highly reliable, safe environments that have complex care requirements and ever-emerging medical sciences and technologies. Nevertheless, serious patient-safety risks are a constant challenge in these environments, especially in the face of multidisciplinary teams using cutting-edge technologies, critical and highly complex medical devices, multiple patient acuities, economic forces that emphasize efficiencies and expediencies, and

Perioperative Clinical Nurse Specialist, Lucile Packard Children's Hospital at Stanford, 725 Welch Road, Palo Alto, CA 94304, USA
E-mail address: chrismith@lpch.org

Perioperative Nursing Clinics 4 (2009) 157–165
doi:10.1016/j.cpen.2009.01.003
1556-7931/09/$ – see front matter © 2009 Elsevier Inc. All rights reserved.

educational challenges strained by regulatory mandates, scarce resources, and a multigenerational work force with varied learning styles. These challenges suggest, even dictate, the use of creative and engaging evidence-based educational modes of simulation that offer multiple opportunities for nurse clinicians to acquire and develop skills in making critical decisions and solving problems, all aimed at furthering patient safety.

THE PROCESS OF LEARNING

Learning is an active, dynamic process that has the potential of transforming the learner. Effective educational strategies must be cooperative, collaborative, and engaging to capture and sustain the attention of new generations of perioperative nurses. The pedagogical and nineteenth-century university models of education are no longer relevant or acceptable in the twenty-first century. Common and accepted educational wisdom tells us that we remember and understand considerably more information when we are actively involved in the process than when we passively watch or hear someone lecture.[1] Adult learning is typically mediated through experience. Consider the alignment of *wise* with *old*. Learning is a process of gaining knowledge through the transformation of experience and logical information with critical-thinking and decision-making abilities integrated into our habits through real-life experiences.[2,3]

Clinical nursing practice is reflected in three distinct yet interrelated and interdependent domains of skills and learning: clinical/technical knowledge, interpersonal (affective behaviors like surgical conscience) skills, and critical-thinking (decision-making) skills.[4] Competence is essential to safe clinical practice and evolves from a foundation of evidence-based perioperative nursing knowledge, as demonstrated in measurable actions and behaviors.[5] Porter-O'Grady[6] describes competence as not about having skills, but about using skills to achieve desired outcomes. The progression of acquiring competency skills has been elegantly described by Dreyfus and by Benner[7,8] as a journey from novice learner/practitioner through levels leading to proficiency and expertise, promoted by concrete didactic education, opportunities for experiential learning, reflective questioning, and paradigm shifts that are manifested in confidence, intuition, global perspectives, and advocacy.

The metrics of educational outcomes continue to remain rather subjective in terms of critically measuring competency. What is the definition of *competent* other than "safe to practice independently in the presence of a strong scrub/circulator partner?" The connection between nursing competency and safe clinical performance has yet to be fully established or adequately clarified.[5] Clinical education today strives to orient staff properly to dangerous devices and patient-safety goals to protect the patient and facility from sentinel events and to accumulate the requisite documentation to protect the institution's staff, unit, and facility from serious regulatory sanction. While institutional staff members may excel at post-tests following in-service programs and have files full of check lists and wallets full of certification cards, they may still fall short in clinical performance, confidence, self-efficacy, and good decision-making during those rare but potentially lethal events that test nerves and the limits of expertise.

GENERATIONAL IMPLICATIONS IN TEACHING AND LEARNING

Today's workplace is a multicultural, multigenerational diverse universe of core values, formative experiences, social expressions, lifestyles, and characteristics that affect the fabric of the work milieu. Much has been written about the learning and motivational needs and styles of the next generations (those born since 1965). These new needs and styles impact work ethics, intergenerational perceptions of the other generation's work ethic, abilities to communicate, and acceptance of technology and change.[9]

These new learners want to be mentored, do not want to be bored, and thrive in team-based learning and work environments. They respond well to frequent feedback, corrective recommendations, and action plans. They perceive themselves as successful and strive to meet expectations. They love to learn and adapt to varied educational formats with technological enhancements and fast-paced interactive fun.[10] Deck[11] emphasizes that this new generation, with its short attention span, learns through interactive sessions of 10 to 15 minutes with brief breaks that offer an unexpected distraction activity. Deck also recommends that educators incorporate physical movement and repetition of critical information while catering to the new generation's learning style preferences of combined seeing, hearing, and doing.

Providing an interactive, structured learning environment for critical components of perioperative education and practice supports and promotes the advancement of the profession and safe patient care. Keeping this valuable, well-educated and technologically literate new generation in perioperative nursing is crucial to the survival of the profession and to the easing of the nursing shortage in the future. This new generation of perioperative nurses truly has the tools and abilities to take nursing to new levels.

SURGICAL SIMULATION AND VIRTUAL REALITY AS A TRAINING MODALITY

Simulation training provides comprehensive learning opportunities in a risk-free environment and promises to prepare learners for the complexities of today's clinical practice. Simulation learning is changing the face of clinical education. Applications include individual skill and team training, confidence building, competency assessment, and rehearsal of crisis management scenarios.[12]

Simulation training is an educational model that strives to create an artificial, or virtual, reality. Virtual reality permits the educator to mimic actual clinical scenarios that provide clinicians with a realistic platform on which to practice the integration of didactic knowledge, assumptions, skills, communication techniques, and collaborative behaviors so as to manage or accomplish a common clinical goal.[12,13] It permits clinicians to learn safely, to practice, and to repeat a skill as many times as needed to gain proficiency, which in turn fosters critical thinking, active learning, confidence building, and professional satisfaction.[14] Simulation training offers many advantages for educators and learners over traditional passive classroom learning (**Box 1**).

THE SIMULATION LABORATORY

Nursing fundamentals laboratories, a foundation of nursing education for the last century, typically use hospital cast-offs and outdated supplies. In the last few decades, newer equipment, nearly lifelike manikins, and, frequently, student volunteers, have been used in attempts to replicate the clinical setting. The ability to simulate clinical reality in the learning environment depends upon the availability of durable and disposable equipment, manikins, models, and simulators.[15]

Durable equipment includes operating room beds, instrument tables, directed energy machines (eg, electrosurgery units, lasers, ultrasonic dissectors), surgical instruments, basins, syringes, lights, positioning devices, and other equipment needed for the selected learning activity. Disposable equipment, devices, and supplies are necessary, as are functioning durable counterparts. Disposable items include electrodes, fibers, catheters, drapes, sutures, disposable laparoscopic instruments, and stapling devices. These items may come from outdated supplies, supplies

---

Box 1
Advantages of simulation training

Develops clinical and decision-making skills without risk

Engages and motivates active learning

Improves performance

Provides immediate feedback

Builds confidence

Builds professional self-satisfaction

Promotes team building and familiarity with other team members

Provides environment for repetition to enhance memory, speed, and psychomotor skill

Integrates best practices into teaching

Promotes testing and development of pioneering techniques

Promotes interdisciplinary communication

Offers role modeling and role development opportunities

Cultivates integration and synthesis of knowledge through reflective thinking

Enables the educator to assume a mentor/facilitator/evaluator role

Provides opportunities to learn from mistakes and discover problems

Demonstrates for learner that, in the perioperative setting, a team working together can accomplish more than individuals working seperately

Re-creates unusual events to determine causative factors

---

contaminated before use, and some purchased or pulled from stock and considered part of the cost of clinical education.

Adding life like manikins, anatomic models, and computerized simulators creates a realistic, controlled clinical platform that assists the learner in acting out skills, reviewing skills, and synthesizing classroom knowledge into practical techniques. High-fidelity manikins are equipped with feedback technology (software and hardware) that can be manipulated by the facilitator to provide a variety of outcomes. High-fidelity manikins have been used for several decades to train cardiopulmonary resuscitation instructors and students seeking Advanced Cardiac Life Support and Pediatric Advanced Life Support certification.

Newer generations of manikins provide hemodynamic parameters on a monitor, breath and bowel sounds, moans, crying, chest movement, palpable pulses, heart sounds, and dysrhythmias. Several models respond to learner interventions, such as cardiopulmonary resuscitation, intubation, and medication administration. These manikins are available as full and partial male or female adult and pediatric models.[13] Higher manikin fidelity provides the learner with more realistic encounters. Lower fidelity manikins are static models, such as the basic cardiopulmonary resuscitation torso or baby manikin. The selection of appropriate equipment, manikins, and models depends on expected learning outcomes, design of simulation activities, and the availability of resources.[15]

Simulation activities may also include the use of other available resources or tools to demonstrate a clinical situation. These may be used in combination with high- and low-fidelity equipment or used alone. Examples of such activities include video games and other kinds of games, role-playing practice, and case studies. These activities sometimes can prove to be effective educational tools when designed and facilitated around clear learning objectives and evaluative end points.

CLINICAL PERIOPERATIVE APPLICATIONS FOR SIMULATION EDUCATION

The perioperative environment, given its interdisciplinary team-dependent care model, its wide use of highly complex technology, and its position in a care-delivery system that depends in large part on human factors, provides rich opportunities to practice, test, investigate, and validate patient-care processes. Simulation applications are appropriate for perioperative education through a continuum of orientation, in-service education, and continuing education (**Box 2**).

The operating room and interventional procedure rooms provide convenient learning laboratories when unoccupied. Educators may design scenarios to address high- or low-volume as well as high- or low-risk procedures or practices, based on the clinical unit's scope of care and the educational abilities, preparation, and skill sets of staff. Simulation offers opportunities to reinforce skills and knowledge. Used nonpunitively, clinical education via simulation nature may result in the staff's validation of its own abilities, increased self-confidence, and enhanced satisfaction as clinicians. Often, preceptors and role models emerge and collaborative relationships develop when staff members work together on a common goal.

Collaborative participation by other, preferably all, perioperative services staff, including ancillary, technical, and clerical staff; clinical students of other disciplines; preoperative and postanesthesia care unit staff; surgeons; and anesthesia staff can promote enhanced interpersonal communication and flattening of the surgical/procedural hierarchy. This happens as everyone learns each other's roles, responsibilities, and scopes of practice, as well as each others' names. This educational and social exercise can enhance the value and depth of the time-out briefing with more collaborative communication. It can also promote the postprocedure debriefing with reflective thinking and expressions of important information, concerns, or suggestions.

DESIGNING PERIOPERATIVE SIMULATION SCENARIOS

A well-designed simulation scenario follows a logical framework of required elements undertaken in a specific order:

1. Identify the learner group, selecting any and every team member who could be involved in the real-life situation. A dynamic scenario involves members of all participating disciplines.[13]
2. Select the educational topic (see **Box 2**). A learning-needs assessment or implementation of a new procedure may guide the decision.
3. Develop the simulation learning objectives that will lead to the desired outcome. Use evidence-based practice guidelines, algorithms, protocols, and references.
4. Describe the elements and characteristics of the planned scenario. A template for designing simulation scenarios may guide the selection of elements (**Box 3**).
5. Determine the fidelity required to provide a successful active-learning setting with the available resources in mind.
6. Identify expected activities needed to demonstrate the desired outcome and achievement of objectives.
7. Identify evaluation method(s).
8. Determine debriefing questions.

Box 2
Perioperative applications for simulation scenarios

Perioperative core competencies (examples)

    Surgical positioning

    Electrosurgery use

    Creating and maintaining the sterile field

    Scrubbing, gowning, gloving, de-gowning

    Radiation and laser safety

    Pneumatic tourniquet safety

    Surgical counts

    Preoperative skin preparation

    Moderate sedation administration

Communication

    Preoperative nursing assessment and interview

    Time-out, preoperative briefing, and postoperative debriefing

    Surgical counts

    Delivering bad news/apologizing for an error

    Hand-off reports

    Conflict intervention/resolution

Emergency response and management

    Sentinel event re-creation and review

    Cardiac arrest/shock response

    Latex allergy reaction

    Malignant hyperthermia crisis response

    Loss of airway/respiratory arrest

    Airway fire

    Operating room fire with evacuation

    Disaster drill: fumes, bomb threat, earthquake, power outage

    Mass casualty trauma triage

Mock surgery scenarios

    New procedure or equipment before first case: robotics, transplant

    New physician

    New multidisciplinary team

    New department/facility before opening

    Patient with transmission-based precautions

---

9. Develop a script using the template or list of required elements. Determine what information each member will or will not know before the start of the scenario. Identify any cues that might drive the scenario to keep it on task (eg, laboratory calls with new results).[16]

Box 3
Sample elements in a template for designing simulation scenarios

Scenario title: Airway Fire

Learner group: four-person surgical team

Expected run time: 15 to 20 minutes

Scenario summary of characteristics: setting, patient, procedure, event

Learning objectives: two to eight (the learner will demonstrate)

Psychomotor skills required before simulation: intubation, circulate for tonsillectomy

Activities required before simulation: review electrosurgical unit safety and fire triangle

Activities expected during scenario: assist anesthesia to extubate/reintubate

Fidelity: manikin, props, equipment, diagnostics available, documentation mode/forms, team roles

Important information related to roles: orientee, staff nurse level IV, angry surgeon

Significant laboratory values: patient has congenital cardiac myopathy

Physician order: turn electrosurgical unit up to maximum power setting

Name of facilitator

Method of evaluation

Debriefing questions

---

10. Set up the simulated clinical scenario.
11. Review each participant's role and describe the objectives without giving too much information that could hinder participants' accurate demonstration of current knowledge and skill. Do not give away the ending.
12. Direct learners to step into their roles by giving a short report. Observe as they interact with the manikin, equipment, and team. Allow mistakes, but avoid progression to a catastrophic outcome.[16]

EVALUATION OF OUTCOMES OF SIMULATION SCENARIOS

After participants complete the scenario, have the learners step out of their roles and relocate to another room to debrief and engage in guided reflection. Evaluation is important to determine if the outcomes are being accomplished. The method of evaluation depends on whether the scenario was intended to be formative or summative.[14] A formative evaluation measures accomplishment and progress toward a goal, provides feedback, and promotes self-reflection by validation of knowledge and skills-acquisition (eg, learning to work as a team member responding to a pediatric code). A summative or summary evaluation occurs at the end of a learning session or specific time frame to measure attainment of learning objectives. This type of evaluation often ends with competency sign off.

Evaluation can be accomplished with observation; checklists; questionnaires; attitude scales; anecdotal notes in a journal, diary, or log; group discussions with consensus agreements on outcome; or any combination of these methods. A facilitator guides the debriefing with planned, probing open-ended questions that direct learners to reflect on the scenario and to make judgments on performance, the validity of assumptions, observations, mistakes and recognition of limitations (eg, lack of equipment, not calling for help, or not delegating), team behaviors, feelings, and where learners believe they did well and not so well.[13,14,17] A video replay of the scenario, often invaluable, may be viewed and critiqued. Debriefing is designed to invite the learner to reflect on personal assumptions and knowledge, to foster new learning, and to validate in a nonthreatening environment.[18] It is not intended to be punitive.

SUMMARY

A 3-year national, multisite, multimethod research product sponsored by the National League for Nursing and Laerdal Medical compared the learning experience of three groups of nursing students. One group collaborated on a paper/pencil case-study simulation. The second group participated in a hands-on simulation with a static, low-fidelity manikin. The third group also participated in the simulation, but did so with a high-fidelity manikin. All three groups used the same simulation case study and participated in a 20-minute, guided reflection session. Members of the high-fidelity group, compared to members of other groups, were more satisfied and confident with their performance and viewed feedback as more important.[19]

Feedback and guided reflection facilitate the critical-thinking, decision-making process. Simulation requires learners to self-discover and to make logical sense of what, why, and how they know. High-fidelity clinical simulation scenarios incorporate more principles of best practices. Learners in such clinical simulation scenarios have the best opportunity to apply and to synthesize knowledge and skills in a realistic and nonpunitive setting that promotes safe and competent practice.

REFERENCES

1. Available at: http://lpc1.clpccd.cc.ca.us/lpc/hanna/learning/activevspassive.htm. Accessed September 20, 2008.
2. Kolb DA. Experiential learning: experience as the source of learning and development. Saddle River (NJ): Prentice-Hall Inc; 1984. p. 20–39.
3. Ulrich L, Glendon K. Interactive group learning: strategies for educators. 2nd edition. New York: Springer; 2005. p. 1–13.
4. DelBueno D, Barker F, Christmyer M. Implementing a competency-based orientation program. Nurse Educator 1980;5(3):16–20.
5. Stobinski JX. Perioperative nursing competency. AORN J 2008;88(3):417–76.
6. Porter-O'Grady T, Malloch K. Quantum leadership: a textbook of new leadership. Sudbury (MA): Jones & Bartlett; 2005. p. 15.
7. Available at: http://209.85.173.104/search?q=cache:rDWKOcytirUJ:azmec.med. arizona.edu/Dreyfus%2520Model%2520of%2520Skills%2520Acquisition.ppt+ dreyfus,+skill+acquisition&hl=en&ct=clnk&cd=1&gl=us. Accessed September 26, 2008.
8. Benner P. From novice to expert: excellence in clinical practice. Commemorative edition. Saddle River (NJ): Prentice-Hall Inc; 2001.
9. Swenson C. Next generation workforce. Nurs Econ 2008;26(1):64–5.
10. Lower J. Generation Y. American Nurse Today 2007;2(8):26–9.
11. Deck M. The latest and greatest ways to teach the television generation of learners. Available at: www.tool-trainers.com/games/0.greatest.html. Accessed September 29, 2008.
12. Saver C. OR business conference in San Francisco. OR Manager 2008;24(7): 24–5.
13. Anderson M, LeFlore J. Playing it safe: simulated team training in the OR. AORN J 2008;87(4):772–9.

14. Jeffries PR, Rogers KJ. Evaluating simulations. In: Jeffries PR, editor. Simulation in nursing education: from conceptualization to evaluation. New York: National League for Nursing; 2007. p. 87–103.
15. Spunt DL. Setting up a simulation laboratory. In: Jeffries PR, editor. Simulation in nursing education: from conceptualization to evaluation. New York: National League for Nursing; 2007. p. 103–22.
16. Childs JC, Sepples SB. Designing simulations for nursing education. In: Jeffries PR, editor. Simulation in nursing education: from conceptualization to evaluation. New York: National League for Nursing; 2007. p. 35–58.
17. Decker S. Integrating guided reflection into simulated learning. In: Jeffries PR, editor. Simulation in nursing education: from conceptualization to evaluation. New York: National League for Nursing; 2007. p. 73–85.
18. Childress RM, Jeffries PR, Dixon CF. Using collaboration to enhance the effectiveness of simulated learning in nursing education. In: Jeffries PR, editor. Simulation in nursing education: from conceptualization to evaluation. New York: National League for Nursing; 2007. p. 123–35.
19. Jeffries PR, Rizzolo MA. Designing and implementing models for the innovative use of simulation to teach nursing care of ill adults and children: a national, multi-site, multi-method study. In: Jeffries PR, editor. Simulation in nursing education: from conceptualization to evaluation. New York: National League for Nursing; 2007. p. 147–59.

Fundamental Perioperative Nursing: Decompartmentalizing the Scrub and Circulator Roles

Carol R. Ritchie, MSN, RN, CNOR

KEYWORDS

- Scrub role • Scrub nurse • Circulating nurse • Circulating role
- Delegation • Communication • Perioperative education
- Patient safety

At one time, operating room nurses always served also as scrub nurses. Today registered nurses predominantly circulate and the scrub role is delegated to surgical technologists. While the registered nurse no longer routinely takes on the scrub role, he or she needs to be comfortable and confident when determining who will "scrub" and then supervising the scrub person. However, many registered nurses in perioperative settings are not experienced in the role of scrub person. To address this problem, Scottsdale Healthcare and collaborators developed a scrub fellowship for registered nurses. The scrub fellowship program teaches experienced perioperative nurses how to scrub on the majority of high-volume procedures in their perioperative services department. Scrubbing increases the perioperative nurse's knowledge about procedures and provides direct experience and appreciation of activities at the sterile field. This gives the nurse greater competence at delegating, a learned skill that requires experience as well as effective communication. Furthermore, The experience in the scrub role improves the nurse's ability to identify and speak up about potential patient safety concerns, and gives the perioperative nurse confidence and competence to supervise the person assigned to the scrub role.

CHIEF COMPLAINT: "WHAT'S GOING ON OVER THERE?"

The patient is draped. The nurse conducts the time-out with the surgical team. An incision is made and the procedure gets started. The surgeon begins requesting retractors, sponges, and instruments from the scrub person. The nurse sits down at the computer to begin charting. There is a steady quiet chatter as the scrub person

Scottsdale Healthcare, 7400 East Osborn Road, Scottsdale, AZ 85251, USA
E-mail address: critchie@shc.org

Perioperative Nursing Clinics 4 (2009) 167–180
doi:10.1016/j.cpen.2009.01.001
1556-7931/09/$ – see front matter © 2009 Elsevier Inc. All rights reserved.

periopnursing.theclinics.com

and surgeon continue their work. The surgeon begins dissecting down to the inner layers of tissue using the electrosurgical unit (ESU). She sets the ESU down on the sterile field and begins using pickups and scissors. The room hums with the sounds of the monitors and a cadence of voices, as instruments are requested. The circulating nurse makes his way around the field to see how things are progressing.

The nurse, an experienced scrub person, looks over and sees the ESU pencil lying on the patient as the surgeon leans over to position herself at a better angle for dissection. The nurse cautions the surgeon, "You're leaning on the Bovie!" Then the nurse says quietly to the scrub person "Please put the ESU in the holster when it's not being used. We had a close call last week because the ESU was left on the sterile field. The drape was burned!"

Would the nurse have been as quick to notice this fire hazard if he was unfamiliar with the scrub role? Would the nurse have spoken up about this safety hazard if he were not directly familiar with common safety measures at the sterile field? This is just one example of a real patient-safety situation. Perioperative nurses who scrub know the multiple safety risks underlying policies and procedures that mitigate those risks. Let us ask the question about the elephant in the room. Perioperative nurses who perform on a regular basis in the scrub role should be able to better demonstrate competence to delegate and supervise this role.

There are very few nursing specialties where the nurse provides direct nursing interventions while concurrently observing and being accountable for the actions of several other team members. The perioperative nurse is often expected to delegate, supervise, and evaluate the activities of other team members working at the sterile field while simultaneously executing immediate directives and interventions in urgent or emergent situations. Such breadth and depth of responsibilities require the ability to think critically and make quick decisions at a moment's notice. The nurse's listening, observing, and anticipating skills must be well honed and finely tuned. The nurse must be constantly aware of what is happening on and off the sterile field and be able to prioritize actions, evaluate interventions, and swiftly adapt to changing circumstances.

The perioperative nurse works in an environment characterized by work-around processes rather than hard-wired engineering processes. Such an environment does not easily accommodate error prevention methods used by industry and in fields employing automated processes, making the nurse's role in ferreting out potential errors more difficult and more important. The operating room environment can also be quite capricious. The circulating nurse is strictly accountable for errors, but when that nurse vigorously raises concerns about potential errors, he or she often faces criticism as being obstructive, annoying, or needlessly fussy.

Whichever way we look at it, the work environment in operating rooms has been notoriously intimidating. Accreditation and government agencies now see a link between preventable adverse patient outcomes and operating room environments that are excessively intimidating or otherwise dysfunctional in some way.[1] Perioperative patient-care settings across the country are examining their cultures of safety and are beginning to swiftly and boldly address problematic behaviors that have the potential to foster medical errors. In many work environments, the consequences of communication mistakes and other errors are normally trifling. But in the operating room, stakes are high, and errors can prove very costly or even deadly. That is why many health care educators, managers, and administrators are urgently seeking hard-wiring methods to improve communication processes and behavior accountability measures to reduce errors. At Scottsdale Healthcare, the scrub fellowship has been implemented as one mechanism to improve teamwork and collaboration in perioperative patient care.

OPERATING ROOM HEALTH ASSESSMENT

The mid- and late 1800s delivered a paradigm change in health care. Florence Nightingale,[2] among a number of pioneers dedicated to caring for the sick, was disturbed by the high morbidity and mortality rates of the sick. She sought better outcomes through changes in and study of the basic care of her patients. Nightingale, a Unitarian, was mindful of biblical health laws, especially with regards to cleanliness. She followed this belief system to establish the basis for patient care, with further explications on healing and health. She studied and wrote about the need for a clean environment, good ventilation, ample light, proper nutrition, warmth, adequate rest, relief from stress and annoyances, separation of infected material, separation of patients with infections, and preventative care for surgical patients. Much of Nightingale's work to improve the environment of care is illustrated in existing perioperative practices.[3]

Nightingale's major focus of care for the surgical patient was prevention. She wrote:

The surgical nurse must be ever on the watch, ever on her guard, against want of cleanliness, foul air, want of light, and of warmth... Nevertheless let no one think that because sanitary nursing is the subject of these notes, therefore, what may be called the handicraft of nursing is to be undervalued. A patient may be left to bleed to death in a sanitary place.[2]

Nightingale eloquently explained the basic requirements for nursing care over 100 years ago. However, these requirements did not supersede care for emergencies threatening life and limb. She expected the use of common sense and judgment.[2] Those same attributes are expected of the perioperative nurse in the 21st century.

OPERATING ROOM HISTORY: ASSISTING WITH SURGICAL PROCEDURES

It is in operative cases particularly that it is most important for a nurse to be conversant with the principles of asepsis and antisepsis, and to understand their practical application...Cleanliness and surgical cleanliness are two different conditions. It is not enough that all appliances should be free from foreign matter perceptible to the eye, not enough that they are spotless and shining, but they must also be absolutely free from any infectious particles, and must be kept so from the beginning to end of the operation.[2]

Nursing practice, as it progressed in the late 1800s and into the early 1900s, provided comprehensive primary patient care. Nurses did not have a specialty designation as they do today. Instead, nurses provided complete start-to-finish patient care and were solely relied upon for surgical procedures.[2,4] Then, when civil and world wars led to shortages of nurses, focused training of operating room personnel took place not only in hospitals but also on the battlefields. At first, registered nurses assumed the scrub role while operating room technicians performed in the circulating role. This continued until 1965 when the roles reversed and registered nurses assumed the circulating role, thereby delegating scrubbing to the technicians.[5,6] This change was based on the nurse's education and ability to assess the patient-care situation, make critical decisions, and knowledgeably supervise the care delivered. Nightingale's reminder about the nurse being conversant with principles of asepsis and even the care of those instruments at the sterile field remains valid, even though the nurse is no longer working predominantly in the scrub role. Thus, the nurse must understand both the role of the circulator, which he or she most frequently performs, and the role of the scrub person, a role less frequently performed by the nurse.

THE OPERATING ROOM'S PHYSICAL EXAMINATION: STAFFING RATIOS OR RATIONING?

While nursing shortages over the years may have affected the way staffmembers were assigned in perioperative settings, the main consideration nowadays in assigning staff is often cost-effectiveness. Salaries consume over 50% of hospital financial resources. Budgets thus become much more manageable when more lower-paid staff members are added to the employment mix. Perioperative leadership teams, in the budget-balancing quest, are faced with the task of maintaining the delicate recommended equilibrium of licensed professional nursing staff members with surgical technologists and unlicensed assistive personnel while also maintaining salaries within established budgetary constraints.[6,7]

A trend that developed in our perioperative department over a period of time was a slight reduction in the registered-nurse/surgical-technologist ratio and the number of positions allocated to registered nurses. This resulted in restricting registered nurses mainly to the circulating role, with only rare opportunities to serve the scrub role. As a result, according to an informal survey, fewer than half of registered nurse staff members are comfortable in the scrub role.

The subsequent reduced number of allocated positions for registered nurses was not solely due to the unavailability of registered nurse applicants for perioperative positions. An analysis of the history of one of the perioperative departments revealed that the imbalance was attributed to budget constraints, a taxing work environment that prompted registered nurses to seek different positions, and subsequent conversion of unfilled nursing positions to positions for surgical technologists.

The perioperative leadership team, heading one of our units with a flatter ratio, has been converting vacant surgical technologist positions to nursing positions, when possible. Our perioperative services leadership team highly values competent and committed surgical technologists and it is not the goal to replace surgical technologists completely. The goal now is to ensure a ratio of 2:1 or 67:33 registered nurses to surgical technologists according to the Association of Operating Room Nurses (AORN) recommendations.[8]

DIAGNOSIS
Imbalanced Skill Mix

Fluidity, flexibility, and efficiency are core characteristics of a nursing presence in the surgical services department. In departments with recommended staffing ratios, managers report a better and more professional working environment, improved team efforts, and efficiencies that make financial goals easier to attain. These managers note that break and lunch assignments are easier to assign and turn-around times are more efficient when a nurse is readily available for these purposes. The scrub fellowship prepares circulating nurses to assume the role of scrub at a moment's notice, thereby contributing to a well-organized and resourceful patient care setting.

The introduction of the scrub fellowship has rekindled interest among perioperative nurses to take on the scrub role and has given these nurses confidence and capability to perform the role well. Once nurses learn the skill, they cherish it and most nurses rarely turn down an opportunity to scrub. Eventually, as the proper ratio of nurses is reestablished in the department, we foresee more opportunities for nurses to participate on the surgical team in the scrub role. We believe that amplification and strengthening of nurse participation in the scrub role will lead to improved teamwork, more effective collaboration, and greater confidence in oversight of the role. The quality of patient care and the promotion of a culture of safety depend, in part, on the ability of the nurse and surgical technologist to efficiently communicate and work together to improve outcomes of surgical patient care.

A crucial issue surrounding staffing ratios is their relationship to patient outcomes. According to AORN's staffing recommendation position statement, several studies have correlated a lower ratio of registered nurse caregivers with adverse patient outcomes.[8-10] While studies of perioperative patient outcomes as they relate to skill mix are difficult to conduct because of so many variables, there are widespread anecdotal reports of concerns with team relationships. Many of these reports mention confrontational discussions with members of the surgical team who are quietly, or not so quietly, uncooperative during the course of usual patient-care routines. Overt or passive uncooperative behaviors undermine patient safety and quality of care. While much research and discussion of imperiled cultures of safety in the operating room focus on uncooperative or disruptive behaviors among physicians and nurses, these behaviors exist among other members of the surgical team, including perioperative nurses and surgical technologists. The question arrises whether nurses who are uncomfortable in the scrub role may be more likely to keep quiet about a concern or questionable practice at the sterile field. Perhaps this may occur because he or she may perceive a lack of credibility to question a practice of which they have no direct familiarity. We suggest that, with nursing competence in the scrub role, the registered nurse will more capably and confidently speak up and raise questions with members of the surgical team.

Even though benefits of reestablishing recommended ratios are loosely linked to outcomes at this point, the institution is moving forward with its plan and the scrub fellowship program. We are confident that nurses who scrub are more watchful and attentive circulators and are more skilled at global thinking. Circulating nurses who develop their skills in the scrub role bring a comprehensive focus to the sterile field and a heightened mindfulness of patient safety.[11]

Reestablishing the recommended ratio of surgical technologists to registered nurses will afford more scrub opportunities for perioperative nurses. It is expected that nurse satisfaction and retention will increase, thereby reducing recruitment, orientation, and training costs. The nurse functioning in the scrub role contributes to comprehensive surgical patient care, bringing perioperative nursing practice to fulfillment with substantial and additional direct patient-care skills at the sterile field.

Delegation of an Unfamiliar Skill

Economic and health care–related financial trends directly and indirectly affect staffing in the operating room, as well as in hospital systems in general. Operating rooms, the revenue-generating machines of hospitals, are continually scrutinized to maintain efficiency and often struggle to function within the budget. Managers are further challenged to maintain staffing levels, comply with regulatory requirements, and meet scorecard metrics, all the while agonizing about preventing medical errors and delivering quality patient care.

The use of surgical technologists and support personnel in the operating room is essential for overall financial health. When nursing shortages required operating room managers to seek viable options to make the most of their existing nursing staff and their budget, more hospitals hired surgical technologists to take positions normally held by registered nurses.[5,6,12,13] State requirements, thus far, have limited surgical technologists to scrub-role functions. Centers for Medicaid and Medicare services still require registered nurses to directly supervise surgical technologists or licenses practical nurses in scrub roles.[14] However, without successful and competent delegation and supervision of delegated tasks, quality patient care comes into question.[15,16]

The ability to make good decisions requires not only knowledge, but also experience. Nurses placed in the circulating role without adequate scrub experience may be lacking the basic foundational knowledge to adequately supervise team members functioning in this role.

A serious question arises when the tasks or skills being delegated are unfamiliar to the person doing the delegating. When this is the case, the recipient of the delegated task may not be receiving adequate supervision to carry out the task safely and completely. Appropriate delegation ensures that the recipients of the delegated tasks are being assigned to another individual with the proper level of training and demonstrated competence.

Nursing practice of assessment, planning, and evaluation of patient outcomes cannot be delegated.[17] However, certain aspects of the plan of care, once it has been devised, can be delegated. What tasks or interventions fall into this category and when? Are the responsibilities of the registered nurse in the operating room limited to performing the preoperative nursing assessment, administering medications, performing counts, documenting, and receiving written and verbal physician orders?

Perioperative professionals and departments have been placed on a slippery slope. AORN states that the scrub role is a delegated function,[9] but many perioperative nurses are not able to efficiently function in the scrub role. Perioperative nurses advocate the need for a circulating nurse in the operating room, yet may be placed in a difficult position when they are expected to appropriately delegate and supervise a role in which they might not be fully competent to perform.[17]

Appropriate delegation of a job function requires knowledge of the delegated function.[18] It also requires the knowledge of delegation responsibilities including oversite or supervisory provision of the delegated role. In our first small group of perioperative nurses participating in the scrub fellowship, only those nurses who had previously completed the in-house residency program for novice perioperative nurses were aware of the scrub role as a delegated function. In that program, delegation is thoroughly discussed. The other nurses who had not attended the in-house residency program as part of their orientation and education as a novice were unaware of their responsibilities to provide oversight of the scrub person.

Delegation of an Unfamiliar Skill: Consequences

When there is a reduced number of nurses of perioperative nurses on staff and a lack of understanding of the key responsibilities in the scrub role, other team members may function independently or in a compartmentalized way. This phenomenon developed into a patent-safety concern within one of our departments with a flatter staffing ratio. The patient-safety issue involved the practice of instrument care and handling at the sterile field.

Instrument decontamination practices deteriorated from established standards over time. A number of elements contributed to the breakdown. Surgical technologists were not thoroughly educated in central sterile processing department practices, perioperative nurses were not involved in instrument care and processing, and the overall process was not hard-wired. Care and cleaning of instrumentation during and immediately following procedures was inconsistent among team members. Wiping instruments with sterile sponges moistened with sterile water during the procedure was infrequent. The surgical technologists, over time, had developed habits outside of recommended practices, and the nurses, not fully familiar with the underlying rationale for keeping the instruments free of blood and body fluids, seemed uncomfortable addressing the concern.

Meanwhile, in the departments in which most of the perioperative nurses have scrub experience, proper instrument care was routinely practiced and there were conscious efforts by the scrub person to keep instruments clean during the procedure. The nurses who scrub in that department understand that preparation for decontamination begins at the point of use and they do not hesitate to speak up about instrument care.

In the department not following standard protocols for caring for instruments at the sterile field, the problem was brought to the attention of the manager and the unit patient care committee. The care and handling of instruments used during the procedure was addressed, a new guideline agreed upon, and processes are being reestablished. The committee addressed the concerns, brought nurses familiar with established practices of professional associations to the discussion table, and set performance expectations for all scrub personnel. Now educational and compliance processes are being hard-wired into the department for instrument care beginning at the point of care. Included as a part of ongoing education is a regular work rotation of surgical technicians into the central sterile processing department.

Poor Communication

It has been 10 years since the legendary 1999 National Institutes of Health study on medical errors.[19] This oft-cited report began the work establishing cultures of safety in health care organizations. In 2000, the Joint Commission reported data on root causes of medical errors. Among the most common causes were discrepancies in communication.[20,21] If delegation is rooted in effective communication, and poor communication is a cited root cause of medical errors, how can we expect quality patient outcomes when we have yet to address the problem of poor communication?

Effective delegation requires communication skills that embody trust, respect, and professionalism.[18] We cannot expect that delegated components of the perioperative plan of care will be communicated and supervised properly, and further expect quality care and good patient outcomes, if the person doing the delegating is not prepared to describe, demonstrate, and evaluate the performance of the delegated task or procedure.

Our health care system is laden with poor communication as evidenced by the Joint Commission's analysis of data on root causes of medical errors.[21] Effective, open, and honest communication is a learned ability requiring interpersonal skill, knowledge, and experience. It is a skill for which many members of the perioperative team have had little formal training, yet one that is an essential and elemental requisite in a perioperative department that strives to create a culture of safety. Exacerbating the issue is the often hierarchical and sometimes intimidating perioperative work environment, addressed in a recent report from the Joint Commission and linked to patient safety and medical errors.[1]

Can a perioperative nurse delegate properly when effective communication skills are lacking? What are the consequences when there are flat staffing ratios that require more delegation and supervision? Do surgical technologists and surgeons understand the tenets of delegation? We may have lists outlining what to delegate, but do we also focus on how to relay the message and to coach staff on building positive relationships and collaboration? Do we expect competence in delegation and ability in nonconfrontational communication of new staff? Considering the rising number of medical errors, the challenge of nursing, surgical technology, and medical education programs should be to incorporate effective communication and discussions of delegation into their curriculum and administrators should require demonstration of this competency from their employees.[12]

Delegation in the Operating Room Today

The joint statement published by the American Nurses Association and the National Council of State Boards of Nursing defines delegation as "the process for a nurse to direct another person to perform nursing tasks and activities." The nurse is accountable for the outcome of the delegated act.[15] The two organizations also agree that the definition of supervision is the "guidance and oversight of a delegated task." Considering this definition, would it be more appropriate to refer to the role of the surgical technologist as a supervised role rather than delegated role? Oft repeated is the dilemma: Since many perioperative nurses are not familiar with the scrub role, how can we fairly hold them responsible for a practice or skill in which they are unfamiliar?

RECOMMENDED TREATMENT: IMPROVE COMMUNICATION AND DELEGATION SKILLS

But in both [hospitals and private houses], let whoever is in charge keep this simple question in her head, (not, how can I always do this right thing myself, but) how can I provide for this right thing to be always done?
—Florence Nightingale

In our institution, which is similar to many others, we have taught novice perioperative nurses how to position a patient, apply the electrosurgical dispersive pad, and open sterile supplies. We discuss how to sterilize instruments and how to prepare one's hands during surgical hand antisepsis. While the list of what we cover is long, we have recently begun to ask ourselves if we have taught them skills to be able to communicate, delegate, supervise, speak up, use the chain of command, ask for help, and identify the right thing to do at the right time in the right way and with the right voice. Even if we review this in the classroom, the real learning comes with practice and experience—both necessary to effective communication, delegation, and supervision.

Preparing perioperative nurses to function at the sterile field in the scrub role is one educational method to develop these essential skills. Working in this role helps the nurse circulator develop confidence, relationships, and credibility; expand knowledge of procedures; and cultivate coordination, organization, and critical-thinking skills.[9,11]

Learning Delegation

Dexterity in delegation requires practice and experience. It also requires a certain amount of interpersonal skill and commitment to the process. Nyberg[5] outlines necessary elements for successful delegation. These elements include trust, engagement and active participation, education and practice, communication, monitoring, and team building, which incorporates mutual respect and courtesy. Additional components, outlined by VanCura,[22] include management support, role competency, appropriate delegation, teamwork, and effective communication.

According to Hall,[13] the proper teaching of delegation requires that an educational component be added to existing nursing curriculum. Education should emphasize the overarching role and responsibility of the nurse for the whole team. The staffing structure, common to the operating room, includes surgical technologists and operating room assistants or nursing assistants. Curriculum related to delegation should include role clarity for all staff members. The nurse, responsible for direct and indirect care by team members, requires education, training, and coaching on how best to work collaboratively with other team members, on interpersonal skills, on skills-based training in conflict resolution, and how best to provide feedback.

How do we teach delegation skills? One method is to begin with practiced situations based on real scenarios. Nyberg[5] gives a number of examples of what verbal communication skills to use when delegating. The most important ingredient in such verbal skills is a positive approach. When language is positive and directed to the desired patient outcome, it comes naturally. When delegation is performed with understanding and respect, mutual trust and teamwork is developed.

ASSOCIATION OF OPERATING ROOM NURSES POSITION STATEMENT ON THE ROLE

The Association Perioperative Nurses (AORN) position statement on the role of the scrub person outlines and describes the importance of maintaining an active registered nurse presence in performing the scrub role.[9] The position statement cogently describes the scope of responsibility of the perioperative nurse in the scrub role, noting the cognitive, behavioral, and technical acumen required in perioperative nursing practice. To achieve desired patient outcomes, AORN believes, as does Scottsdale Healthcare, that an active registered nurse presence in the scrub role assists the perioperative nurse in appropriately delegating portions of the patient's plan of care.

RECOMMENDED PROCEDURE: ESTABLISHING A SCRUB FELLOWSHIP OF THE OPERATING ROOM

Our perioperative services leadership group endorsed and gave full financial support to the rollout of the scrub fellowship program for registered nurse circulators. The scrub fellowship program is designed to provide perioperative nurses, inexperienced in the scrub role, direct scrub experience in a variety of relatively uncomplicated procedures.

This 8-week program was based on knowledge of the perioperative nurse's role and incorporates nursing interventions applicable in the scrub role. Six registered nurse circulators participated in the program developed in collaboration with Delaware County Community College and its perioperative nursing faculty.

The program has identified three desired outcomes: (1) to heighten the nurse's awareness of key responsibilities and functions of the scrubbed member of the surgical team, (2) to increase the ability to anticipate the needs of the scrub person, and (3) to establish the perioperative nurse as qualified to delegate and supervise the scrub role.

Other benefits of the program include:

- Providing nurses with opportunities for more variety in daily assignments, thereby, enhancing job satisfaction
- Giving nurses greater credibility, resulting in more respect from the surgical team
- Helping nurses, through the experience in the scrub role, gain better appreciation of the challenges of the scrub role
- Improving team relationships within the department
- Promoting perioperative practices that meet higher standards of professionalism

BACK TO SCHOOL
Schedule and Curriculum: Planning Meeting

In November 2007, perioperative clinical educators at Scottsdale Healthcare collaborated with those at Delaware County Community College and its perioperative nursing faculty in designing the class schedule and curriculum plan for the scrub fellowship. The planning team settled on the basic schedule and program topics as outlined in **Table 1**.

Selection Process

Selecting nurses for the program was simplified for the first group of fellows. Members of the planning team needed to secure commitment from the managers, announce the class to the perioperative nursing staff, evaluate the completed fellowship application forms, and make the selections, within a short time. The managers also needed to meet with the scheduling supervisors to ensure that those selected for the fellowship would be allotted education time for classroom work as well as the clinical scrub time.

The application form included several questions and requested a brief essay that included reasons for wanting to learn the scrub role. We also prepared a worksheet for the managers to help them in the selection process. That worksheet, which covered questions listed in **Box 1**, included phrases commonly used in evaluations, thereby giving the manager objective and subjective tools to assist in the applicant-review process. One recommendation made for the selection process was to include a requirement for certification. It remained a recommendation rather than

Table 1	
Basic schedule and program topics for scrub fellowship	
Schedule	**Topics**
Week 1	
Day 1	Introduction and history of perioperative nursing Patient- and family-centered care Introduction to the scrub role
Day 2	Sterile technique; safety; accountability; adaptability Scrub, gown, glove, draping, counts (lecture) Luncheon with Associate Vice-President, directors, and managers Afternoon skills laboratory (scrub, gown, glove)
Day 3	Continuation of scrub role lectures Phases of surgery Afternoon skills laboratory
Week 2	
Day 4	Instrument processing and sterilization Skills laboratory
Day 5	Hemostasis, wound closure, wound healing Skills laboratory
Week 3	
Day 6	Minimally invasive surgery; instrumentation, procedures, and safety
Day 7	Patient safety issues; medications, universal protocol, fire prevention, specimens
Week 4	
Day 8	Conflict management Delegation Specialty equipment as requested Individual presentations; case studies
Day 9	Group exercise Final examination Luncheon

Box 1
Worksheet questions to help managers in the selection process for scrub fellowship
Is the candidate certified?
Does the candidate have basic scrub skills in some services?
Does the candidate practice according to professional standards?
Does the candidate show genuine enthusiasm for perioperative nursing?
Is the candidate a "self-starter?"
Is the candidate supportive of departmental goals?
Does the candidate demonstrate professional behavior?
Does the candidate practice according to the vision and values of Scottsdale Healthcare?
Does the candidate volunteer for additional projects?
Is the candidate a team player?

a requirement because we did not want to dampen enthusiasm with an overabundance of stipulations for participation; however, this particular recommendation may be upgraded to a requirement for future fellows. We asked those interested in the first scrub fellowship for a commitment to seek certification.

In consideration of the short time frame, the maiden voyage of this class required some latitude in qualifications. We also needed to ensure enough participants to make the fellowship worthwhile. The selection process depended ultimately upon the managers and their budgets. Managers reviewed the objective and subjective information from the application forms, and then, with their own assessment using the worksheet evaluation tool, selected those they believed were the most appropriate candidates.

Participant demographics varied. Nurses participating in the fellowship represented an assortment of experiences. Four participants had previously taken part in the perioperative residency program for novice perioperative nurses. These particular nurses had received basic scrub training and had scrubbed for 3 weeks during their residency program. They also had the benefit of learning from perioperative educators and of communication skills acquired from working in the operating room. However, they had scrubbed infrequently since the residency program.

One of the participants explained that she never quite "caught on" to the scrub role during her original perioperative residency, relating that it was too overwhelming at the time. The two remaining nurses were experienced operating room nurses upon hire but without any formal or consistent scrub experience. They had scrubbed in the past, but rarely and for very minor procedures. One of the participants related his past experience with loading and passing sutures. He had never been instructed on handing the needle holder and, when this was covered in class, he was quite enlightened when he realized he had been passing the suture backward all of this time.

Curriculum Building and Remodeling

Topics from portions of the Scottsdale Healthcare in-house residency program for novice perioperative nurses were used in building the curriculum for the scrub fellowship. Modifications, including higher-level lectures, were added. It was important during the implementation process to consider the expertise of the nurse participants in the design and ongoing remodeling of lecture content. The nurses who participated in the program were experienced circulators. The content and teaching methods needed to incorporate adult learning styles and the nurses' existing clinical expertise.

The nurses had been exposed to the scrub role in the past but felt intimidated and lacked sufficient confidence to volunteer to scrub.

The initial outline, a modification of the in-house perioperative residency program, provided the infrastructure to the scrub fellowship program. Lesson plans for each class day were modified slightly as the program progressed. The final content enhanced the breadth and depth of existing knowledge and tested participants' critical thinking. Specific skill review and competency assessment sessions were conducted in a simulated laboratory setting. These topics are listed in **Box 2**.

Extra Credit

What we learned

The results of the first scrub fellowship program were modest, as we realistically expected. We learned from the fellowship evaluations that nurses who learned to scrub felt more at ease and proficient in the scrub role and were more comfortable speaking up as circulators when there was a problem at the sterile field.

We also were pleasantly surprised with unanticipated outcomes. Several surgical technologists spoke about their desire to enroll in nursing school or seek certification. Many of our surgical technologists participated as preceptors during the fellowship. They were excellent preceptors and enjoyed being part of the educational process. This renewed their desire for learning as they saw the growth in their team members.

Immediate, 4-month, and 6-month evaluations

The evaluations were comprised of a rating system of one to five, one being the lowest score. We asked the fellows to rate the content and the instructors. The initial evaluations were as expected. Fellows requested more time with hands-on practice using specialty equipment, such as drills and fixation devices. The class content was

---

Box 2
Topics for specific skill review and competency assessment sessions

Organization skills

   Mayo stand

   Instruments required for each case

   Bowel technique

   Efficiency

   Safety

   Anticipation (before case starts)

   Specialty draping

   Paying attention to the field (concentration when there are so many distractions)

Instrumentation skills

   Power drills

   Contents of trays

   Laparoscopic trays

Suture skills

   Passing suture (no pass zone)

   Closure requirements

sufficient but the class times were held on Thursdays and Fridays, normally very busy times in the department. This often created a conflict with staffing. Overall, however, the participants valued the program and believed that this type of program was very important to the perioperative nurse's ability to anticipate, respond to, plan for, and participate in events taking place at the sterile field.

The 4-month evaluations revealed that the fellows were being assigned to scrub less frequently. In the 6-month evaluations, three of the six nurses revealed that they had not scrubbed in at least 2 months.

The clinical educators discussed the situation with the managers and scheduling supervisors, asking for a renewed commitment to this program. Modifications are being made to the next fellowship program to ensure commitment and accountability from the supervisors and the participants. The perioperative nurses participating in the next program will be required to document a specific number of hours within a set number of weeks to receive their completion certificate. We also are planning to schedule a follow-up class 3 months post–fellowship completion to review accomplishments and challenges. The staffing supervisors will be requested to assign a nurse in the fellowship or a nurse who has completed the fellowship to scrub whenever possible, thereby helping those competent in the scrub role to maintain their skills.

SUMMARY: SCRUBBING IS "FUNNER"

Satisfaction and fulfillment comes from the nurses' presence in the scrub role. Whether removing a lesion or repairing broken bones resulting from a horrific blunt trauma vehicular crash, nurses who scrub welcome the variety that this role brings to their workday. But, regardless of the situation, the nurse who scrubs also appreciates the magnitude of performing focused nursing care during one of the most vulnerable times in a patient's life.

William Duffy,[11] in an article about the scrub role, eloquently explained how his experiences as a surgical technologist prepared him to be a circulating nurse. Scrubbing teaches anticipation, organization, and efficiency, he explained, and circulating nurses who have served in scrub roles have a heightened awareness of these core skills, which can lead to improved patient outcomes.

The scrub fellowship is one mechanism to foster development of nursing competency in the scrub role. The value of this type of program may be difficult to measure in concrete patient outcomes data. However, most experienced nurses describe scrubbing as both a valuable and an enjoyable part of their work. The consensus among nurses completing the scrub fellowship is that perioperative nursing is much "funner" when they have the opportunity to scrub. When words like *fun* and *enjoyable* are used to describe one's work, intent to stay is bolstered and a sense of well-being is created. These attributes, in and of themselves, lead to harmony in the workplace. That is an outcome that deserves to be copied!

REFERENCES

1. Joint Commission on the Accreditation of Healthcare Organizations. Sentinel event alert: behaviors that undermine a culture of safety. Available at: http://www.jointcommission.org/SentinelEvents/SentinelEventAlert/sea_40.htm. 2008. Accessed August 3, 2008.
2. Nightingale F. Notes on nursing: what it is, and what it is not. Harrison & Sons; 1860. Available at: http://www.books.google.com. Accessed August 10, 2008.

3. AORN. Recommended practices for environmental cleaning in the perioperative setting. In: Reno D, editor. Perioperative standards and recommended practices; 2008. p. 375–89.
4. Weeks-Shaw CS. A text-book of nursing. New York: D. Appleton and Company; 1894. p. 13–4.
5. Nyberg DB. Successful delegation skills enhance patient care. AORN J 1999; 69(4):851–6.
6. Phippen ML, Applegeet CJ. Assistive personnel in the perioperative setting: changing the paradigm. Semin Perioper Nurs 1992;1(2):103–20.
7. Murphy EK. Unsubstantiated assumptions about unlicensed assistive personnel obscure the challenge of delivering quality patient care. AORN J 1995;62(1):8–10.
8. Association of Perioperative Registered Nurses (AORN). Position statement: operating room staffing skill mix for direct caregivers. In: Reno D, editor. Perioperative standards and recommended practices; 2007. p. 413–4.
9. AORN. Position statement: statement on the role of the scrub person. In: Reno D, editor. Perioperative standards and recommended practices; 2008. p. 407.
10. Shamian J. Skill mix and clinical outcomes. Can Oper Room Nurs J 1998;16:36–41.
11. Duffy WJ. The importance of keeping our hand in the scrub role. AORN J 2004; 80(5):817–9.
12. Krainovich-Miller B, Sedhom LN, Bidwell-Cerone S, et al. A review of nursing research on the use of unlicensed assistive personnel (UAP). J N Y State Nurses Assoc 1997;28(3):8–15.
13. Hall ML. Policy implications when changing staff mix. Nurs Econ 1998;16(6): 291–7, 312.
14. Centers for Medicaid and Medicare Services (CMS). Hospital conditions of participation: surgical services. Available at: http://edocket.access.gpo.gov/cfr_2004/octqtr/pdf/42cfr482.51.pdf. Accessed August 3, 2008.
15. National Council of State Boards of Nursing (NCSBN). Joint Statement on Delegation American Nurses Association (ANA) and the National Council of State Boards of Nursing. Available at: https://www.ncsbn.org/Joint_statement.pdf. Accessed August 10, 2008.
16. Marshall M. The use of unlicensed personnel: their impact upon professional nurses, patients and the management of nursing services. Nursing monograph 2006. Available at: http://www.ciap.health.nsw.gov.au/hospolic/stvincents/2006/nursing%20monograph2006.pdf. Accessed August 17, 2008.
17. NCSBN. Working with others: a position paper. Available at: https://www.ncsbn.org/Working_with_Others.pdf. Accessed August 10, 2008.
18. Cohen S. Delegating vs. dumping: teach the difference. Nurs Manage 2004; 35(10):14 18.
19. Institute of Medicine (IOM). To err is human: building a safer health system. Available at: http://www.iom.edu/Object.File/Master/4/117/ToErr-8pager.pdf. 1999. Accessed August 10, 2008.
20. JCAHO. 2009 National patient safety goals. Available at: http://www.jointcommission.org/NR/rdonlyres/40A7233C-C4F7-4680-9861-80CDFD5F62C6/0/09_NPSG_HAP_gp.pdf. Accessed August 4, 2008.
21. JCAHO. Sentinel event alert: operative and post-operative complications: lessons for the future. Available at: http://www.jointcommission.org/SentinelEvents/SentinelEventAlert/sea_12.htm. 2000(12). Accessed August 17, 2008.
22. VanCura BJ. Five key components for effectively working with unlicensed assistive personnel. Available at: http://findarticles.com/p/articles/mi_m0FSS/is_n5_v6/ai_n18607524/pg_4. 1997. Accessed August 17, 2008.

The Need for Educated Staff in Sterile Processing—Patient Safety Depends on It

Rose Seavey, RN, BS, MBA, CNOR, CRCST

KEYWORDS

- Sterilization • Decontamination • Processing • Instrumentation
- Disinfection • Storage

In a rapidly changing world, technology alters almost every aspect of life, and its effects are quite evident in the perioperative setting. A technology explosion has enabled noninvasive or minimally invasive procedures to be performed in myriad settings, including the operating room (OR), ambulatory surgery centers, cardiac catheterization units, endoscopy suites, physician's offices, and radiology departments. Whether these procedures use high-tech surgical devices (ie, robotics) or more common, everyday surgical instruments, reprocessing these items safely and effectively is a vital part of every surgical/invasive procedure. Patient safety depends on surgical instruments that are properly cared for, effectively reprocessed, and ready to use (ie, instrument readiness). These measures require knowledgeable, responsible people and a workplace that facilitates effective and efficient processing. Surgical instrument reprocessing is the responsibility of both the OR and the sterile processing department (SPD).

Without the SPD, today's perioperative nurses would be unable to deliver high-quality, safe, and cost-effective health care to patients. Nursing shortages, budget limitations, advances in sterilization technology, and the need to stay abreast of ever-changing recommended practices for reprocessing surgical instruments have intensified the need for perioperative professionals to collaborate with sterile processing professionals. Surgical case volumes rise each year, and OR managers and educators have the responsibility of orienting inexperienced nurses as quickly as possible.[1]

In addition to training nurses, educators must ensure that those taking care of surgical instruments are knowledgeable about the processes in the SPD. This article explores the need for a comprehensive training program for staff assigned to reprocess surgical instrumentation.

Seavey Healthcare Consulting, Inc., 6810 W 52nd Place, Arvada, CO 80002, USA
E-mail address: rose@seaveyhealthcareconsulting.com

Perioperative Nursing Clinics 4 (2009) 181–192
doi:10.1016/j.cpen.2009.01.002
1556-7931/09/$ – see front matter © 2009 Elsevier Inc. All rights reserved.

periopnursing.theclinics.com

HISTORY OF THE STERILE PROCESSING DEPARTMENT

In 1933, the American Sterilizer Company developed the first steam sterilizer that allowed temperature to be measured with a thermometer. This development began the modern era of sterilization. Credit for the birth of sterile processing, however, goes to the American College of Surgeons. This association first suggested standards for the handling of surgical dressings and the centralization of handling and preparation of all surgical supplies in one department. Hence, the Central Supply (CS) came into being as a distinct unit.[2]

Historically, most surgical supplies and instruments were prepared by OR staff. Between cases or at the end of the scheduled day, the OR staff would go to the "workroom" to wash and wrap instruments, sponges, gloves, dressings, drapes, and other supplies, and then send them to CS to be sterilized. Most OR nurses did not know what "SPD" meant. They knew only that the CS department in the basement housed the supplies not stocked in the OR, sterilized items too large to be processed in the OR, and offered overflow space for supplies that surgery could not store. In the past, the OR could function more or less independently, because surgery had become a profit center and revenue leader that could afford to pay OR nurses to perform these essentially non-nursing tasks. No more! As surgical case volumes increased, nursing shortages became acute, innovative technology advanced exponentially, and the bottom line became critical to institutional survival, hospitals of necessity decided to delegate surgical reprocessing duties to CS and SPD.

PATIENT SAFETY

The Association of periOperative Registered Nurses' (AORN) Position Statement on Patient Safety states

> The safety of patients undergoing operative or other invasive procedures is a primary responsibility of the perioperative registered nurse. Registered nurses form a professional bond with patients, who place their physical and emotional well-being in the hands of registered nurses and their surgical colleagues and who believe that the care provided will be safe and effective. The patient/caregiver bond is founded on the patient's trust in the registered nurse and the surgical team. Protecting the patient and promoting an optimal surgical outcome further strengthens that bond.[3]

When one talks about "surgical colleagues" and the "surgical team," one now must include the instrument reprocessing staff. Even though staff members are not physically at the surgical table, the products it produces have a critical effect on patient safety. The instrument processing staff therefore play a very important role in concert with the surgical team and should be held as accountable for patient safety as the OR nurse, the surgeon, the anesthesiologist, and the scrub technician.

Given this vital role, staff that reprocess surgical instruments and pick case carts must be knowledgeable, experienced, and held responsible for their part in patient safety. Today's sterile processing demands critical thinking skills, because surgical instruments are more complicated than ever. The reprocessing staff deal with exceptionally complex devices with many delicate, multifaceted parts and long, narrow, intricate lumens. The more complex an item is, the more difficult it is to clean and sterilize. These new devices come with very specific and sometimes difficult reprocessing instructions that require absolute compliance to ensure sterilization and safe patient care. In the future, if not today, facilities no longer will be able to afford to staff the department with entry-level SPD employees.[4]

EDUCATIONAL NEEDS

Employees performing sterile processing duties (eg, cleaning, decontamination, instrumentation preparation, packaging, sterilization, storage, and transportation of sterile items) must be trained properly to execute these tasks efficiently and effectively. This training is not exclusive to those assigned to SPD but also includes nurses and technicians working in the OR. This discussion pertains to the education of SPD staff responsible for reprocessing surgical instrumentation.

ORIENTATION

To meet the need for knowledgeable, qualified SPD staff and to ensure the safety of patients and employees, all SPD staff must go through a comprehensive training program. This orientation should be a formal, structured program that is consistent and standardized. Depending on the services provided by the SPD, orientation can take from 3 to 18 months.[2]

A standardized orientation program helps ensure that all employees are taught the same information using the same processes. One of the most effective ways to achieve a standardized orientation program is to have each trainee assigned to a knowledgeable and experienced preceptor who follows a consistent orientation program. The preceptor monitors the employee's training and serves as a mentor for the new employee.

Preceptors should be knowledgeable about how to be a preceptor. They should have proven competencies in what they are teaching and how they teach it. If a facility has more than one person in orientation at a time, it may hold formal classes. Competencies should be validated with return demonstrations, proving that the trainee understood the information and is capable of performing the duties.

SPD staff process many critical items used directly on patients, and therefore, just as in the OR, it is paramount to have a dedicated educator for SPD staff orientation. In some facilities SPD staff education may be the responsibility of the perioperative educator. Larger facilities may have a designated SPD educator. For the program to be successful, upper-level management should be involved and supportive.

Adults sometimes seem to learn new things faster experientially, rather than through visual or auditory training. Being engaged in the learning involves risk and susceptibility. Having the trainee perform a return demonstration for every new task learned is a helpful evaluation tool. Indeed, experiential learning may be key to successful adult learning. A comprehensive education and orientation plan should include, but not be limited to, the following subjects:

- Basic medical terminology
- Basic human anatomy and physiology
- Basic microbiology
- Infection prevention and control
- Regulations, standards, and recommended practices
- Surgical instruments
  - Handheld surgical instruments
  - Powered surgical instruments
  - Endoscopic instruments
  - Resources for surgical instruments
- Cleaning and decontamination processes
- Instrument preparation and tray assembly
- Decreasing errors in instrument sets

- Sterile packaging
- Sterilization and/or disinfection
- Sterile storage

BASIC MEDICAL TERMINOLOGY

Knowledge of basic medical terminology helps SPD professionals understand the importance of their roles and responsibilities. Understanding medical terminology also helps improve communication between OR and SPD staff and increase job satisfaction.

Because most medical terms come from Greek or Latin, the best way to understand their meaning is to break words down into their root elements. Knowing common roots, prefixes, and suffixes will help the staff members analyze and remember medical terms. The SPD staff also must know and understand common abbreviations used for surgical procedures.

Health care facilities frequently offer classes in medical terminology. If schedules permit, such classes may a good alternative to teaching medical terminology in the SPD. These classes can be helpful for new SPD staff and also serve as a review for experienced staff. These classes also can be broken down into small units and used as in-services for the entire department. Posting a medical "term of the day" in the lounge as a review or learning opportunity also can keep staff involved as active learners.

BASIC HUMAN ANATOMY AND PHYSIOLOGY

SPD staff are responsible for assembling and reprocessing surgical instruments and equipment as well as for picking surgical case carts. A basic knowledge of human anatomy, physiology, and cell biology helps staff understand the importance of completeness and accuracy in their work. This basic knowledge also can help staff appreciate policies and procedures and the rationales for them and provides a structure for performing their tasks in an efficient and competent manner. This education should cover basic anatomy and physiology (cells, tissues, and organs) as well as an introduction to the body systems, because this information constitutes the underlying building blocks for staff's understanding of the key mission of thorough, effective, and efficient reprocessing.[5]

Using basic pictures or diagrams of each system helps adult learners visualize how systems work. Posters in the department showing the muscular/skeletal system and vascular system can be a valuable resource for the SPD staff. These posters can be helpful tools in understanding particular surgical procedures.

BASIC MICROBIOLOGY

SPD professionals need a good and current understanding of basic microbiology to protect patients, the environment, themselves, and their co-workers. SPD technicians need to be aware of conditions that favor microbial growth. They should be introduced to the identification and classifications of microorganisms and to the chain of infection and modes of transmission.[6] Understanding basic cell structure and how cells live and grow enables SPD technicians to appreciate better their key role in preventing and controlling infection.

INFECTION PREVENTION AND CONTROL

Every SPD professional plays an essential role in infection prevention and control, and understanding infection and its effective prevention and control should be part of the initial orientation. In addition, every SPD employee should attend an annual review on infection prevention and control, preferably given by the infection prevention and control expert in the SPD facility.

Every course on infection prevention and control should include a discussion of the importance of proper hand washing, the requirements for hospital-issued scrub attire, appropriate use of personal protective equipment (PPE), the Occupational Safety and Health Administration (OSHA) blood-borne pathogens standard(s), hospital-acquired infections, and principles of asepsis. This training also should cover environmental concerns such as physical design, temperature, humidity, and air exchange requirements, the separation of decontamination and clean areas, sterile storage requirements, traffic control, workflow, and work-area cleanliness.[7]

REGULATIONS, STANDARDS, AND RECOMMENDED PRACTICES

The responsibilities of SPD require that all SPD personnel know many regulations, standards, and recommended practices. A regulation is mandatory and is required by law or regulatory body. A standard is considered an established norm determined by authority, research, and/or theory. Standards are not required by law but are considered best practices. Recommended practices are built on sound principles or practice, scientific data, and expert opinions.[2]

Some of regulatory agencies with which the SPD staff should be familiar are the Environmental Protection Agency, the Food and Drug Administration, OSHA, and local state health departments.

The Association for the Advancement of Medical Instrumentation (AAMI) develops standards for sterilization and reprocessing in the health care setting that then are approved by the American National Standards Institute, Inc. (ANSI). "Compliance with AAMI standards and recommended practices is strictly voluntary, and their application is solely within the discretion and professional judgment of the user of the document unless they are adopted by a regulatory authority, in which case it is the regulatory authorities' responsibility to enforce compliance."[8]

Further, some of the most important recommended practices for sterile processing are written by AAMI, AORN, the Association for Professionals in Infection Control & Epidemiology, Inc., and the Society of Gastroenterology Nurses and Associates.

SURGICAL INSTRUMENTS

Health care facilities have a huge investment in surgical instruments, an investment that must be preserved and protected by careful handling, appropriate use, proper cleaning, disinfection, and sterilization, all of which help extend the useful life of surgical instruments. SPD staff responsible for the care and handling of these devices need to know how the devices are made and used. Surgical instruments can be broken down into three major categories: handheld, powered, and endoscopic. An emphasis on understanding these categories and their distinctions will make the learning process easier and faster for new staff members.

Handheld Surgical Instruments

For handheld surgical instruments, SPD technicians need to know the basic functional names (forceps, scissors, hemostats, needle holders, and retractors), their structures (jaws, box locks, shanks, ratchets, and finger rings), grades (floor grade and surgical grade), their functionality (grasping, cutting, suturing, retracting, occluding, transmitting light, conducting electrical impulses, dissecting, aspiration, and probing), and their composition (stainless steel, chrome, titanium alloy, brass, sterling silver, or copper). Instruction should include how to check for functionality as well as for sharpness and damage. SPD technicians also need to know how to maintain handheld surgical instruments and be aware of any special handling needs, such as disassembly or lubrication.[9]

The training process also includes the action that should be taken if a damaged instrument is found and information about available facilities and the procedure for repair or replacement. Many facilities attach nicknames to certain instruments. This practice should be discouraged, because it too often causes confusion and frustration. If a facility nevertheless chooses to use nicknames, it is helpful to use the proper name of the instrument on the inventory list, followed by the nickname in parentheses.

Powered Surgical Instruments

Powered surgical instruments are complex instruments. The processing of instruments powered by an electric motor, compressed gas (pneumatic), or a battery is more intricate than the processing of handheld devices because of the complexity, size, and design of powered devices. Training in this area should include proper hand washing of the instrument, inspection for damage, including the power cords, and proper preventive maintenance, such as lubrication in accordance with the original equipment manufacturer's (OEM) written instructions for care and handling. OEMs often recommend extended sterilization exposure time for powered instruments because of the complexity of the inner parts of these instruments and the oil-based lubricants commonly used. Each OEM user's manual should be readily available for the SPD technicians to review.

Endoscopic Instruments

Most facilities have a wide variety of flexible, rigid, and semi-rigid endoscopes (scopes). Scopes, especially flexible scopes, are very expensive, require exceptional handling, and are challenging to reprocess. Flexible scopes have long, dark, and narrow lumens that pose a reprocessing challenge because they are not directly accessible. Therefore they are extremely difficult to clean. In addition, if the lumens are not thoroughly dried, any moisture will promote bacterial growth.

Each type, make, and model of scope has specific processing issues such as disassembly, channel cleaning, and the need for high-level disinfection versus sterilization. Given the complex nature and design of scopes, anyone responsible for reprocessing them needs extensive specialized training. Training in the care and handling of scopes should include how to care correctly for each specific model, according to the OEM's instructions. The SPD technician responsible for reprocessing these scopes should know where to find the user's manual, should be required to review each manual, and should be instructed to follow the exact procedure given for each specific model of scope.

Resources for Surgical Instruments

Cleaning and decontamination processes

The AAMI defines "cleaning" as the removal of contamination from an item to the extent necessary for further processing or for the intended use.[10] Decontamination is one of the most critical steps in breaking the chain of infection and disease. Decontamination is the process that allows safe handling of reusable items by employees who are not wearing PPE.[11]

Decontamination is a two-step process. The first step is cleaning, manually, mechanically, or by automatic cleaning. The second step is a disinfection process that can be either thermal or chemical. Decontamination is seen as the most important step in the reprocessing cycle, because items cannot be sterilized properly if any bio-burden is present. Therefore, all items must be meticulously cleaned and disinfected before they can be sterilized.

The training objectives for cleaning and decontamination should include, but are not limited to

- A description of all decontamination functions
- Facility-approved policies and procedures for all methods of decontamination of reusable products
- Identification of employee health and safety considerations (eg, the importance and appropriate use of PPE as related to OSHA regulations)
- Guidelines for the selection and use of available cleaning and decontamination processes
- Cleaning processes: presoaking; rinsing; sorting; disassembly; special attention to channels, hinges, and joints; and correct placement of instruments (ie, heavy items on bottom, with box locks open)
- Manual cleaning methods
- Automatic equipment used in the reprocessing of medical devices (ie, instrument washers, cart washers, ultrasonic cleaners, and automatic endoscope washers)
- OEM written recommendations for special cleaning (manual vs. mechanical cleaning, leak testing, lubrication and/or inspection of electrical cords and plugs)
- Facility policy on transportation of contaminated items
- Importance of maintaining a clean work environment

Instrument preparation and tray assembly
Preparing instruments for sterilization has many critical steps; among them are inspection, inventory, assembly, and wrapping. A standardized written procedure for assembling instruments sets and trays helps ensure the consistency of each set. Training in instrument preparation and tray assembly should include but should not be limited to

- The requirement for comprehensive inspection to ensure cleanliness, proper functioning, sharpness, and alignment of each device
- The need for items to be free of corrosion, rust, burrs, pitting, nicks, and cracks
- Specific organization of sets
- Protection for delicate and sharp instruments
- Hinges and box locks must be open
- Instruments with multiple parts should be disassembled unless OEM instructions state otherwise
- The need for lubrication or other specific considerations according to the OEM recommendations
- The importance of following the inventory list for each set
- The preparation of miscellaneous items, including syringes and items with lumens
- The facility procedure for replacing missing or broken items

Decreasing errors in instrument sets
Accuracy is an important part of customer satisfaction and is extremely important with surgical instrument sets. Errors in instrument sets also affect costs by potentially delaying surgery, and checking the instrument set is an essential part of instrument readiness in the OR. Checking for error patterns is the first step in troubleshooting instrument set problems. What are the common errors? Are there missing instruments? Are there dirty instruments in sets? Are any instruments broken and in need

of repair? Are the wrong instruments being put into trays? Are there specific trays that seem to have errors? Are the SPD technicians repeating the same mistakes? Collecting these data and having them available for review can help determine where to start to improve accuracy.[12]

If the SPD has a computerized bar code tracking system, this type of error data can be accessed easily; it is a much harder to track such data manually. Tracking the types and recurrence of errors, however, will provide real and useful data, instead of anecdotal reportage, which is of little use. Once the data are available, the process can begin to determine where errors happen and recur. One should start with basics. Have staff members undergone proper training? Does staff have the resources to complete assigned tasks (eg, are there backup instruments)? Are nicknames used instead of actual instrument names? Do staff members know what to do if instruments are missing or broken? Are the instrument inventory lists complete and accurate, or is it assumed that staff know the lists? Reducing errors should be a quality improvement opportunity for getting staff involved. Ask the SPD technicians what the hardest sets are, what needs clarifying, and what resources they need.[12]

Outcomes can be improved by additional training, broadening and updating inventory lists, creating a database of digital pictures, and using videos, decision trees, and diagrams. If sets are exceptionally difficult, in-service training by the instrument manufacturer's representative(s) may be helpful. If errors occur or recur in specific sets, one can ask the OR specialty service leader to meet with SPD staff to share information and answer questions in a collegial fashion.[12]

Sterile packaging
Packaging systems are used to ensure the integrity of the sterilized contents and permits aseptic delivery of contents. Basic packaging procedures include peel pouches and woven (reusable), nonwoven (disposable), and ridged containers. It is important for SPD staff to understand when and how to use each sterilization packaging method. Considerations should include the size and weight of devices being sterilized.

SPD staff also must learn proper packaging techniques for each category of packaging materials. In addition, they should understand which packaging is appropriate for each type of sterilization method. The importance of air removal, sterilant penetration, the ability to dry instruments effectively, the ability to maintain integrity, the need for aseptic presentation, shelf life, proper closure techniques (sealing tape or locks), and identification labeling should be stressed. If reusable textiles or ridged containers are used, the staff must understand the essentials for proper cleaning, reprocessing, and maintenance of both kinds of containers.

Manufacturers of packaging devices also offer educational in-services. Health care facilities should take advantage of these opportunities to set up an annual packaging review class for all SPD staff.

Sterilization and/or disinfection
Sterilization is a process used to render a product free of microorganisms. Disinfection is a process that kills pathogen organisms by chemical or physical means. Items to be disinfected should be categorized as critical, semicritical, and noncritical, according to the Spaulding classification system. The Spaulding classification, developed in 1968 by Earl Spaulding and adopted by the Centers for Disease Control, categorizes the way items should be processed, depending on the intended use.[1]

SPD staff responsible for reprocessing must understand the difference between sterilization and disinfection, including high-level, intermediate-level, and low-level disinfection. Understanding the nature of a device and the way it is used helps determine the level of reprocessing necessary.[13]

Sterilization Sterilization is the validation process used to render a product free from viable microorganisms.[10] There is no such thing as "almost" sterile. Therefore, facilities must require that knowledgeable people perform sterilization activities. Staff responsible for sterilization must, at a minimum, know and understand

- Principles of sterilization
- Types of sterilization performed
- Different categories of medical devices and specific sterilization methods
- Parameters of all sterilization processes
- Mechanical, chemical, and biologic monitoring systems
- Proper sterilizer loading techniques
- Causes of wet packs
- Steps involved with a sterilization recall process
- Documentation necessary for proper lot control and tracking
- Safety precautions associated with each method of sterilization

Disinfection Disinfection is the process that kills pathogenic and other micro-organisms by physical or chemical means.[10] Education in performing disinfection activities should include basic information about the types of chemicals used in health care facilities such as quaternary ammonia compounds, chlorines, phenolic compounds, alcohols, glutaraldehyde and orthophthaldehyde, and thermal disinfection. The importance of following OEM written recommendations and the chemical manufacturers' instructions for dilution, contact time, and expiration dates should be stressed. In addition, education should cover where to find and how to use each of the Material Safety Data Sheets for each chemical used in SPD.

It is essential that SPD staff be familiar with each device being disinfected so members can ensure that all channels and lumens are cleaned completely and that the disinfectant can reach all areas of the device.

Sterile storage

Proper storage requires that all sterile products be maintained and stored in a way that guarantees sterility until the product is used. When educating staff about the significance of sterile storage, the SPD professional should teach

- The definition of shelf life
- Conditions that can compromise the sterility of a package and its contents
- Basic storage systems
- Requirements for environmental controls and cleaning protocols used in sterile storage areas
- Proper stock rotation
- How and when to use sterility maintenance covers
- Proper handling and transportation of sterile items

Resources

Professional associations offer many valuable resources such as training manuals, standards, and guidance documents, all of which are routinely reviewed and updated. These resources can be used as essential educational tools to improve surgical instrument reprocessing training, education, and practice.

The association of perioperative registered nurses AORN's well-known mission is to promote safety and optimal outcomes for patients who undergo operative and other invasive procedures by providing practice support and professional development opportunities to perioperative nurses. AORN collaborates with professional and regulatory organizations, industry leaders, and other health care partners who support its mission.[14] AORN's Web site is www.aorn.org.

Some years ago, AORN established a specialty assembly (SA) for perioperative leaders who manage or interface with CS, SPD, and purchasing departments. The Sterile Processing/Materials Management SA builds enduring bridges between OR nurses, SPD personnel, and materials management personnel. The purpose of this specialty assembly is to provide and to promote a dynamic collegial network, serving as a forum for communication, identifying and exploring patient care issues, addressing current trends and issues, and promoting specialized education program ming. More information about this assembly is available at http://www.aorn.org/Community/SpecialtyAssemblies/SpecialtyAssemblyGroups/SPMMSA/.

International association for health care central service materiel management The American Society for Healthcare Central Service Professionals and the International Association for Healthcare Central Service Materiel Management (IAHCSMM) merged in September 2007. These combined professional groups are recognized nationally and internationally for providing premier training and technical manuals. The IAHCSMM'S mission is "To provide the members of the Association and health care facilities with organized educational opportunities, professional development, a forum for information exchange, and member services in response to member identified needs and priorities; and to represent Central Service Materiel Management in the professional community." The organization can be found online at www.iahcsmm.org.

Association for the advancement of medical instrumentation The AAMI is a primary source of consensus and timely information on medical instrumentation and technology. It published the excellent reference work, *ST79:2006 Comprehensive Guide to Steam Sterilization and Sterility Assurance in Health Care Facilities*. Sterile processing professionals sometimes refer to this guide as the "sterilization Bible." To develop consensus documents, the AAMI uses committees that include representatives from the medical device industry, government representatives, academic scientists, and individual experts. In addition, major contributors to the development of AAMI-recommended practices for hospital sterilization have been and are OR nurses, sterile processing and infection control professionals, and others with clinical experience. The AAMI can be found online at www.aami.org.

Certifications Two professional certification programs are available for Sterile Processing/CS. They are offered by IAHCSMM and the Certification Board for Sterile Processing and Distribution, Inc. (CBSPD). The CBSPD's stated mission is "To promote and encourage high standards of ethical and professional practice through a recognized, credible credentialing program that encourages the competency of personnel performing sterile processing and distribution activities." CBSPD can be found online at www.sterileprocessing.org

Both these organizations offer certifications in many areas and at many levels (eg, CS technician, supervisor, manager, instruments, and ambulatory setting). Many publications on surgical instrumentation are available.[15]

Another sometimes-overlooked resource is instrument order catalogs from the various instrument OEMs. These catalogues usually are given to the facility at no cost. It is also a good idea to include manufacturers' representatives in the training for complex and/or complicated sets. These representatives have an investment in making sure anyone handling these sets is familiar with them, knows how they are used, and is aware of any special processing requirements.

SUMMARY

SPD plays a significant role in patient safety. Increasing demands are being placed on its staff because of developing technology, more complex sterilization parameters, and heightened monitoring needs. Therefore, health care facilities need to develop comprehensive orientation and training programs for staff responsible for the reprocessing of surgical instruments. Training must be provided by knowledgeable and experienced preceptors. Programs should include all aspects of reprocessing duties as well as basic medical terminology, anatomy, and physiology, microbiology, and infection prevention and control. Orientation, ongoing education, accountability, scrupulous adherence to regulations/standards/recommended practices, and enthusiastic support from upper-level management are essential to a successful SPD professional training program.

REFERENCES

1. Spry C. Introduction. In: Sullivan K, editor. Essentials of perioperative nursing. 3rd edition. Sudbury (MA): Jones and Bartlett Publishers; 2005. p. iii, 31.
2. Chobin N, Evans C, Japp N, et al. Roles and responsibilities. In: The basics of sterile processing. 1st edition. Kenilworth (NJ): Backer Printing, Inc.; 2006. p. 2–14.
3. Association of periOperative Registered Nurses. Position statement on patient safety. In: Standards, recommended practices and guidelines. Denver (CO): Association of Perioperative Registered Nurses, Inc.; 2007. p. 398–400.
4. Swanson S. Shifting the sterile processing department paradigm: a mandate for change. AORN J 2008;88(2):241–7.
5. American Society for Healthcare Central Service Professionals. Human and anatomy and physiology. In: Training manual for health care central service technicians. 4th edition. San Francisco (CA): Jossey-Bass; 2001. p. 22–23.
6. International Association for Healthcare Central Service Materiel Management. Microbiology for central service. In: Central service technician manual. Chicago: International Association for Healthcare Central Service Materiel Management; 2007. p. 60–4.
7. International Association for Healthcare Central Service Materiel Management. Infection prevention and control. In: Central service technician manual. Chicago: International Association for Healthcare Central Service Materiel Management; 2007. p. 99–112.
8. Larrick K. Top 10 things every healthcare professional should know about the Association for the Advancement of Medical Instrumentation (AAMI) standards. Managing Infection Control 2006;6(3):86–8, 95.
9. American Society for Healthcare Central Service Professionals. Surgical instrumentation. In: ASHCSP instructor's guide: training manual for health care central service technicians. 4th edition. Chicago: American Society for Healthcare Central Service Professionals; 2003. p. 165–8.
10. The Association for the Advancement of Medical Instrumentation. Comprehensive guide to steam sterilization and sterility assurance in health care facilities. ANSI/AAMI ST79; 2006. p. 7, 9, 18.

11. American Society for Healthcare Central Service Professionals. Decontamination. In: Training manual for health care central service technicians. 4th edition. San Francisco (CA): Jossey-Bass; 2001. p. 67–68.
12. Lind N. The quest for quality. Infect Control 2008;8(7):80.
13. Association of periOperative Registered Nurses. Recommended practices for high-level disinfection. In: Conner R, editor. Perioperative standards and recommended practices. Denver (CO): Association of periOperative Registered Nurses, Inc.; 2008. p. 305–6.
14. Association of periOperative Registered Nurses. AORN mission and values. In: Conner R, editor. Perioperative standards and recommended practices. Denver (CO): Association of periOperative Registered Nurses, Inc.; 2008. p. 8.
15. Tighe S. Instrumentation for the operating room: A photographic manual. 7th edition. St. Louis (MO): Elsevier Mosby; 2007.

Index

Note: Page numbers of article titles are in **boldface** type.

A

Acute coronary syndrome, simulator scenario for, 106–107

Adult learning, 158

Advanced practice registered nurses, 113, 115, 117–119

Advocacy, 81–82

African-American students, **121–129**
  in associate degree program, 125–128
  in baccalaureate program, 122–125

American National Standards Institute, Inc., 185

AORN. *See* Association of Perioperative Registered Nurses.

Asepsis, 80–81. *See also* Sterile processing department.

Assessment, in associate degree program, 91

Associate degree, **87–95**
  curriculum for, 90–93
  framework for, 87–90
  observation experience in, 93–95

Association for the Advancement of Medical Instrumentation standards, 185, 190

Association of Perioperative Registered Nurses
  on scrub role, 175
  orientation courses of, 108
  Patient Safety position statement of, 182
  sterile processing resources from, 190

Audiovisual aids, in internship program, 151

C

Caring interventions, in associate degree program, 91

Case studies, in internship program, 152

Catheter, intravenous, insertion of, simulator scenario for, 107

Central Supply, 182

Certification, for sterile processing, 190–191

Christiana Care Health System, perioperative internship program of, 141–155

Circulating nurse, duties of, 167–168

Cleaning, in sterile processing, 186–187

Clinical decision-making, in associate degree program, 91

Clinical nurse leader, 113–115

Clinical nurse specialist, 113, 115, 117

Collaboration
  in associate degree program, 91–92
  in simulation education, 161

Commission on Collegiate Nursing Education, 114

Perioperative Nursing Clinics 4 (2009) 193–199
doi:10.1016/S1556-7931(09)00040-0
1556-7931/09/$ – see front matter © 2009 Elsevier Inc. All rights reserved.

Moving?

Make sure your subscription moves with you!

To notify us of your new address, find your **Clinics Account Number** (located on your mailing label above your name), and contact customer service at:

E-mail: elspcs@elsevier.com

800-654-2452 (subscribers in the U.S. & Canada)
314-453-7041 (subscribers outside of the U.S. & Canada)

Fax number: 314-523-5170

Elsevier Periodicals Customer Service
11830 Westline Industrial Drive
St. Louis, MO 63146

*To ensure uninterrupted delivery of your subscription, please notify us at least 4 weeks in advance of move.

Printed and bound by CPI Group (UK) Ltd, Croydon, CR0 4YY

03/10/2024

01040441-0012